# BodyArt Cookbook

## PERFORMANCE NUTRITION PROFESSIONALS RELY ON

# Tanya Lee

bodyartcookbook.com

First Printing, October 2000 (BodyArt Cookbook for Physique Transformation)
2nd Printing, September 2001
3rd Printing, September 2005 Version 2.0 (Fitness Food Cookbook)
On-going printing, 2006-2007, continuous edits
        May 2006 Version 2.1 (Body Transformation Cookbook)
        February 2007 Version 3.0 (BodyArt Cookbook)
        May 2007 Version 4.0
        October 2008 Version 5.0

Cataloguing in Publication Data
Tanya Lee
BodyArt Cookbook
Includes Index
10 digit ISBN 0-9687769-0-6
13 digit ISBN 978-0-9687769-0-2

Published and distributed by www.bodyartmotion.com
Printed by
Blitz Printing AB, Canada
Lulu Press North Carolina, USA


Cover Photo: Tanya Lee by Ken Balaz
Back Cover Photo: Tanya Lee by David Ford  www.davidfordphotography.com

Nutritional information for recipes based from USDA National Nutrient Data Base.

**Disclaimers**
The hardest weight to lose is usually the last 10-30lbs, this system has proven effective for this
goal. This program has worked for Tanya and many of her clients as the testimonials and her titles
adequately indicate. Still the objective truth is that it may not produce similar results for you for
various reasons given each individual has a unique body composition, experiences, demeanor/dis-
position, and values/lifestyle and challenges (emotional-rational, cultural-financial) which requires
a unique adaptation/dosage.

This program in no way should be used as a substitute for consultation with your doctor(s). You
should not consider any presented material by Tanya Lee or BodyArt Motion to be the practice of
medicine or to replace consultation with a physician or other medical practitioner. Tanya Lee
and BodyArt Motion are providing you with information in this consulting work so that you can
have the knowledge and can choose, at your own risk, to act on that knowledge. You are urged
to be aware of your health status and to consult health professionals before beginning any health
program, including changes in dietary habits.

# A Creative Combination For The Conscious Cook!

The search for simple but sensational nutrition has never been easier. BodyArt Cookbook provides readers with wholesome recipes, time efficient solutions and a well-being of body and spirit!

If you are an athlete or interested in achieving goals related to fitness and healthy eating then BodyArt is an exceptional tool. Packed with useful insights, this little gem is a must for the bookshelf.

Developed with a real food attitude there is nothing complicated about this cookbook. Symbols are smartly used to identify recipes by several key objectives - time is one way of selecting appropriate meals to make, as is carbohydrate content and how well a prepared dish will travel!

The research and nutritional details add substance where other cookbooks fall short, making this a resource of knowledge and taste. The authors flavor for flare is evident not only in her spirited writing style but also in the combination of ingredients that line the pages.

A truly refreshing presentation of real food with enticing titles to excite the appetite. BodyArt Cookbook will make you want to get back in the kitchen and enjoy eating healthy!


Inga Yandell

Editor-In-Chief
Bare Essentials Magazine
B.E. A Woman Of Action - Australia

## Oxygen Women's Fitness Magazine USA

The BodyArt Cookbook is a massive collection of simple, convenient, healthy meals. There isn't a fitness athlete out there who wouldn't get their money's worth!

## BodySport Magazine Canada

No matter if you are a competitive athlete or just interested in some recipes to help you eat a little cleaner and healthier, this book is a 'must buy' for everyone that needs a break from boring diet food.

## Jason Dooms Day - Pro MMA Cage Fighter

BodyArt recipes have helped me power through my long work days and training regimen. Tanya makes cutting weight feel effortless! I've never felt better before or during a fight.

## Fatima Kusch - Pro Fitness Model

I am the owner of Blessed Bodies Fitness. FAME Pro Fitness Model Athlete, FAME/WNSO Judge, Certified Trainer, and Registered Sports Nutrition Advisor. For a long time I have looked for a recipe book that works with the foods that I eat for fitness modeling competitions - this one fit perfectly! My "everyday clients" are finding this book to be a very useful tool in helping them come up with new ideas to stick to their food programs.

## Shauna Sky Romano - World Champion -Skeleton

Thank you to Tanya Lee for a wonderful, simple plan that WORKS for everyone. Even those of us with challenges like Celiacs disease (both my daughter and I). Our household eats a mainly vegetarian diet, so it is invaluable for us to have meal options which contain no animal products, but still provide the protein we need!

## SamiTe' - Pro Dancer and Yoga Teacher

This is a fabulous treasure designed for people with specific fitness goals, everyone would appreciate it's clear, concise, and simple approach to a healthful/mindful diet.

## Scott McDermott - Author Speaker Tri-athlete

People always want healthy food that is easy to cook and fast. I realized what a challenge it was to create a truly great, truly different cookbook. When I read Tanya's BodyArt Cookbook, I decided I did not need to do a cookbook. Hers is exactly what I would want to create. Her book is brilliant! It is full of amazing recipes with the breakdowns of all the things you would want to know. After all, why reinvent the wheel?

## Leah McKinnie - Figure Model Champion

People often ask me for advice on getting fit and leading a healthy lifestyle, well I would like to reveal one of my secrets to all of you. The BodyArt Cookbook has fantastic recipes that anyone can appreciate. Nutrition is 90% of the battle, so I strongly encourage you all to check it out.

## Angie Schumacher - Personal Trainer

I am a Certified Personal Trainer and manager of the website womensdietandfitness.com . I absolutely love this cookbook, not only because the majority of the meals are very quick, but they are also very effective! I have lost 6% body fat using this cookbook. I recommend and promote BodyArt Cookbook on my blog, my website and also to my friends and family! This is one cookbook that I was finally able to see results by using!

People pick up this book for different reasons, but it's usually one or more of the following:

- learn to control body weight
- control blood sugar and balance moods
- sculpt muscles like an artist
- increase athletic performance
- balance energy levels
- eat more whole food
- or to just look toned.

Yes, this book can help with all these things.

# body acceptance and objective awareness

Our culture seems to be set up in such a way that an individual's worth is dependant mostly on how they look and/or perform as compared to a Hollywood/Olympic standard.

We are living in a time where self-worth is at an all time low, while information is at an all time high. There are gurus, luscious advertisements, and always another study to tell us what is good and what is bad. When our worth becomes inevitably lower, everyone else's advice naturally begins to sound better than our own.

When you want to change because you're trapped by the panic to get out of a body that is not perfect (by whatever standards you're using to gauge), you make yourself vulnerable to the many tasks of the multi-billion dollar body image mass market.

The new mantra now used as an attempt to counter mass self-esteem trauma executed by "create problem, sell solution" profiteers, seems to be "accept your body the way it is". The problem with this phrase is that no matter the intention, the message is often perceived as "accept that you are less-than". Many people feel that "accepting your body" means to stop the pursuit of fulfilling your potential and to surrender to self-defeating habits.

Acceptance does not mean to stifle desire to work on your body art project. It means to work with what you have been given, not against it. I believe it's essential to view our bodies with as little harsh judgement as possible - to see it for exactly what it is with both weaknesses and attributes. This creates the foundation of your unique flavor and form. Counter to some beliefs, the body is not designed to be an identical replica of an ideal template. And Eve was not likely a super model.

Where the word *acceptance* can often throw a bucket of water on the fire of desire to grow and have you chasing your tail for nebulous reasons as to *why* you feel uncomfortable in your body - the concept of objective awareness feels like a rooted starting point to a rewarding journey.

• Be aware of how your body feels and looks each day.
• No need to judge as good/bad, perfect/not perfect...just observe.

Your body is a lifetime partner. Connect with what *you* see as beautiful and what *you* feel as contentment.

# BOOK CONTENTS

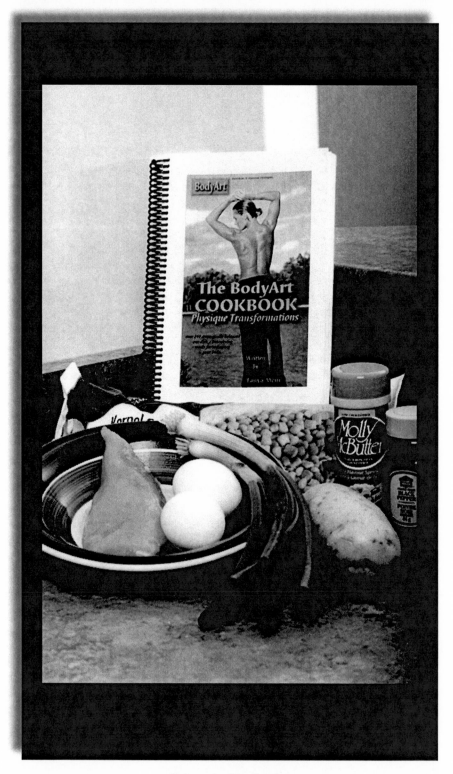

Photographer Terry Goodlad

# COOKBOOK INSPIRATION

Originally, this book was my binder full of recipes during a very busy time in my life.

My early twenties were filled with ambition! I was competing at the national level as a bodybuilder and fitness model when I became a new wife and step-mom, bought my first house, and had a full-time job as a prison guard. In my "spare time" I was planting foundational roots for BodyArt as well as my husbands Mixed Martial Arts School.

I was determined to figure out a way of fitness-eating that was simple, accurate and didn't consume a lot of time. I couldn't see myself eating the same thing day after day, unlike many of my fellow athletes who would drain a can of tuna for lunch and knaw on a dry chicken breast for dinner. If I was going to make this happen, I needed it to be enjoyable with room for creative freedom.

It's important to receive the right information. It is also just as important to focus on how you apply that information. Do you become the diet or does the diet become you? Do you become the lifestyle or does the lifestyle become you? This is the base from which the original BodyArt strategy was built.

When I was crafting my "binder of recipes", BodyArt consisted of private consultations in my living room coaching 1-on-1, 12-week body transformations. Sometimes I would bring my 'secret binder' to meetings and would often make copies of recipes to give to my clients. The meals were so helpful, that they started offering me money for access to my whole binder. A year later, the first *BodyArt Cookbook* was published. It has since shipped to countries across the planet mostly on word-of-mouth merit.

Within five years, I had left my secure government job. BodyArt blossomed to become a beautiful studio with a full schedule of classes, BodyArt certification courses, athlete performance programs, and online consulting across the globe. The BodyArt team has now helped thousands of people achieve personal goals.

In 2004, I was inspired to pursue deeper philosophical roots related to the whole mind-body-soul transformation process, so I chose to take my show on the road, pilot against the wind and the tide of success. I needed solo time to dive into new experiments and explore first hand how the body really is our true home. A series of publications based on my findings and my journey started with this newest version of the *BodyArt Cookbook*, another book called *Alignment Secrets,* and *PowerAlign* - an interdisciplinary movement system for safe and effective training.

Necessity is the mother of invention and this cookbook went through a rewrite to include a "how to use it" section, new foods, vegan/vegetarian recipes, mobile meals on bare bones budgets and more.

## Small town stocky farm girl turned stage-body champion!
The grazing method of eating changed the way I live and strengthened my connection to food and how large it's role actually is in energy balance, weight control, body appearance and muscle recovery.

A stocky tomboy my whole life, I grew up playing power sports and was always training for something. It was rarely a challenge to workout, but no matter what diet I tried I couldn't shake the stocky farm girl figure. Then I found the grazing method of eating 5-6 small macro-nutrient balanced meals every couple hours. Eat more to shed fat - could it be true?

I didn't change my workouts at all and after just three months of grazing I experienced an incredible body change. I had rid of my excess bodyfat and voila...I had muscles! The Body Artist was born. I spent the next ten years in the tunnel of my new found passion. I've taken my body to the edge and back through various vantage points - each time reconnecting yet a deeper layer to the importance of balance.

# THE FOUNDATION

**It's an art to create the body you want to live in.** It doesn't just happen because you want it to happen and if you force it to happen, it will back fire. The process is simple, but layered. There is no need to introduce complicated nutrition formulas if you have not mastered the foundation.

- **Eat every three hours.**
- **When you think you are just about full, stop eating.**
- **Eat more lean protein, veggies, fruit and nuts.**

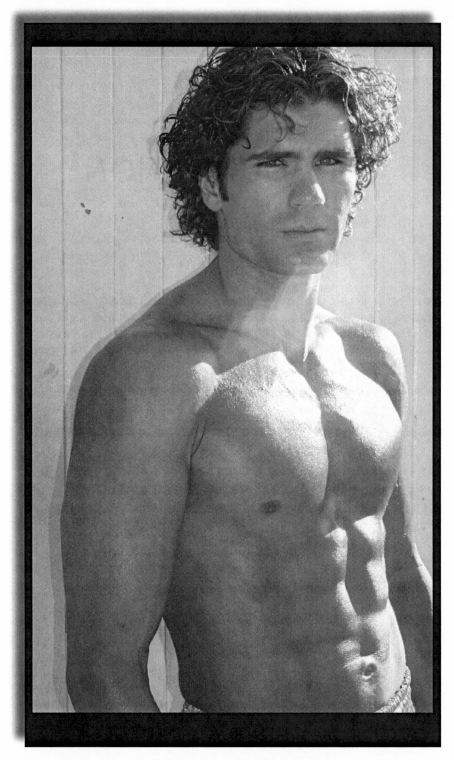

Jason Dooms Day.  Pro MMA Cage Fighter.  Team BodyArt.  www.jasondoomsday.com

# CLARITY & FRAMING
## what we can assume

I used to think cooking was a real drag. Every recipe I tried to follow had at least one ingredient I didn't have in my kitchen and some complicated five step preparation method. By the time I finished reading the directions, I was so hungry that I just ended up eating something pre-packaged.

In my college days, cooking consisted of Ichiban, mac & cheese, microwave pizza pops, and toasted waffles. For anything else, I had to call Mom for directions.

The cooking methods in this book are simple, not gourmet by any means - yes, this book is for the kitchen rookie. From this point on, we are eating for what our body needs. It's about how to create a complete grazing style meal in minimal time when you don't have all the perfect fancy ingredients.

**We can start by assuming** that you are reading this book because you want to feel good about the process of amplifying how you look and feel. We can assume that you either desire to have sculpted body, had it and lost it, or have it and want a fresh perspective on how to sustain it that is perhaps simpler/easier or more natural.

This cookbook has a unique organization of meals to simplify your fat-burn, muscle-fuel project. In it, I focus on foods that can accent your training, meal planning, time management, cooking and eating. I will also briefly cover how to design your food structure according to your current body and goals.

In order to maintain the simplicity of this book, the focus is on whole food. I do not cover micronutrients/vitamins/minerals/hormones or supplements. This food strategy assumes that your body's systems are balanced (we have to start somewhere) and can adequately signal your body to metabolize excess bodyfat. If you eat from this cookbook 80% of the time and you are challenging your body with strength building exercises that make you sweat and breathe deep and you are still not burning fat and/or fueling muscles, you may want to consider the possibility of a biochemical imbalance which you will want to address before relying on any diet to help.

As for body sculpting and performance enhancement supplements, I suggest experimenting with basic natural food strategies for at least a year before attempting to add anything else. Too-many-supplements can create imbalance and lead to panic attacks, mood swings, lack of patience, skewed rationale, and an array of low-grade symptoms we might typically ignore. If you implement too many things all at once, how are you to ever know what intervention to map to the result?

I am not here to dictate what is good or bad for your body. I am here to open some doors so that you may be able to see for yourself what benefits you, what builds the body you want, and what aligns with your lifestyle/values. Your body journey is personal and there just may be more to your unique journey than anyone can have the answers.

When working with clients, I suggest guidelines for nutrition/exercise that I feel may advance their body sculpting journey, but they are often progressive makeover steps tailored to what they are currently doing rather than a complete lifestyle overhaul. The body flows well with sustainable progression. Small changes and baby steps will produce optimum returns on your investments of time/focus/energy.

When it comes to discovering your food strategies the ball is ultimately in your court. One-size-fits-all solutions are a joke. The best advice I can give you at this point is to know your goals and be willing to test different things out – taking what works for you and moving on to the next. It may be helpful to take some time and write down how you want to look, feel, move and express yourself. Then head toward one of these goals and let the rest of your goals become values that you prefer not to sacrifice along your path.

For example let's say your goals are to look like a warrior with radiant skin, feel strong, move like a tiger and express yourself with relaxed confidence. You find a food plan that is designed to get your body lean and muscular. You are three months into a committed food discipline and your body is starting to look great, but you are losing strength and you got a bad case of stinky gas. In this case, the plan is helping you with your body shape goals, but with the GI reaction you are forced to sacrifice one or more of your other values. Not only is your tiger strength sacrificed, chances are your confidence levels may not be that high walking around in a cloud of lethal fumes. At this point, you may want to switch something up or book a nutritional consultation.

The idea is that grazing every couple of hours on one of these balanced BodyArt meals will aid the body in its journey to build, repair and supply the body with a steady stream of energy.

Although nutrition is a huge part of body sculpting, we are going to assume that you are exercising adequately. These meals are designed for athletes, active bodies, dancers, yoga students, fighters, weight lifters, etc. and those looking to transform their shape through challenging their muscles during workouts. In this book, I do touch on some exercise suggestions, but you may want more specifics as to alignment and optimization which are outlined in another book, Alignment Secrets (details in back of this book).

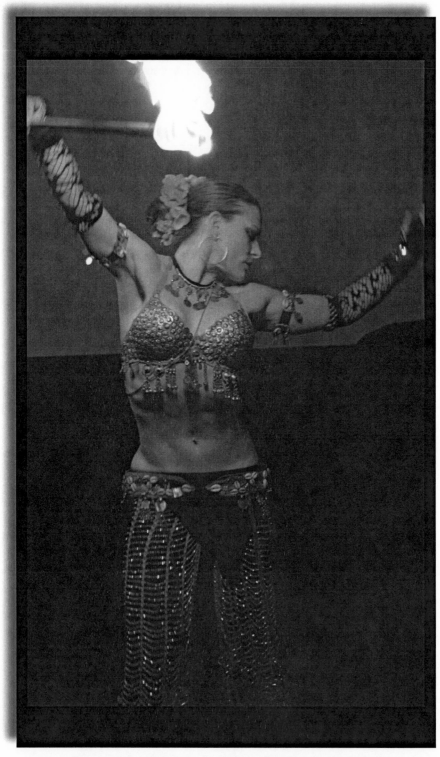

Tanya Lee 2008. Blazing Butterfly Firedance. Live Photo by John Gordon.

# GRAZE WITH PROTEIN
## battle-tested for active bodies

---

graze like livestock : pack your meals!

---

Each meal has a macronutrient (protein/carbohydrate/fat) combination designed for "grazing" every three to four hours throughout the day. The unique organization of this cookbook is based around the fact that to burn fat and fuel muscle one must consume adequate amounts of lean quality protein throughout the day.

In this book I have presented the most common protein sources used in body sculpting (lean chicken, eggs, lean beef, fish, dairy, protein powders, beans). Once you have chosen a protein source then the meal options are varied depending on the type of natural carbohydrate and fat source. This method allowed me to assemble my own recipes into hundreds of well-rounded simple meal ideas.

The grazing strategy may be best understood if you breakdown metabolic concepts into fire concepts. Fire transforms matter and your digestive system is like a fire engine. The word metabolism is used to describe the rate at which your body converts fuel to energy. Placing small to medium size logs and kindling consistently on the flame will keep the fire burning steady with a healthy glow. If you place a whole bunch of big fat logs in the fire all at once, chances are you are going to smother it. The goal is to enjoy the benefits of steady heat - like engineers shovel coal on a steam locomotive.

The technique of grazing has proved successful time and time again not only for athletes and body sculptors, but also for those who just want to lose weight or who have health challenges such as low-metabolism or unstable blood sugar.

## why these meals are organized by type of protein.

I was competing as a top national-level bodybuilder and then as a figure model. I had many clients, owned a pilates/yoga studio and was a wife/step mom all at the same time. I wanted to be able to compete and also do all the other things in my life.

My family and I preferred cooked/prepared meals from natural sources, grains, vegetables, meats, etc. So to not constantly be in the kitchen I needed good time management skills, a well orchestrated plan and well measured recipes.

How did I do it? I started to observe my eating patterns and noticed a significant pattern that each meal is built around a base of quality protein. Some meals include a protein source with grains, some with veggies, some include fat and some don't – but the constant is always protein. It just made sense to organize a booklet not around breakfast, lunch, dinner – but rather by protein food type (i.e. chicken, fish, beef, dairy, etc). This was an added bonus for one who likes to eat a breakfast meal for dinner!

Organizing this book by protein type has helped tremendously with meal planning. Today, I just look in my kitchen to see what protein source I have most available or feel like eating. If it is beef, then I flip open to the beef chapter and choose what looks good at that time. This book really does make this style of eating less stressful and more sustainable.

## macronutrient ratios

After choosing protein type, the next step to building a meal is to add carbohydrates and fats. So it just made sense to make every meal in this cookbook per a one-dish style that contained all three macronutrients in a ratio that promotes fat-burn and muscle-fuel. It would just be a pain in the butt to find a protein recipe and then go find a veggie recipe and then go find a rice recipe, etc.

As I'll explain later, to focus on just calories without prior focus on food discipline, food type and macronutrient ratios may not be the best path for your body sculpting project. This is what you commonly see in the old school weight loss groups – count your calories – where it doesn't matter what type of food you eat. If your goal is an athletic shape – this won't cut it.


## the backbone of these meals

Like noted earlier, there is no one-size-fits-all path to body sculpting. However, there are general nutritional guidelines for fat-burn muscle-fuel that are universal which form the backbone of this book.

BodyArt recipes are created from and inspired by:

- scientific principles of fat-burn and muscle-fuel tangibly proven over decades by top athletes, bodybuilders and fitness models
- health enhancing foods inspired by wholistic practices

This book is separated into meals with and without meat. Combining fundamentals from both vegan and traditional meat-eating programs, this book bridges both worlds and introduces ways for those who aim to reduce an absolute reliance on volumes of extreme meat without sacrificing the protein needed to sculpt the body.

The format had to be flexible for a large number of different bodies and lifestyles. This may be the one rare occasion, a yogi and a bodybuilder might eat from the same cookbook!

Since most North Americans are finding themselves in a race against time, I had to use ingredients that were easy to find in any regular grocery store. The intention was to keep it simple and accessible. You will not see a lot of foreign ingredients you can't pronounce. And even if there is a "strange" or uncommon ingredient, it is explained in simple terms.

To help lessen the amount of times we surrender to fast-food, I needed to create an array of simple and quick meal variations using natural whole foods. To make the meals count for fitness and body sculpting, each recipe had to be scientifically calculated with optimum macronutrients. This was my creative challenge!

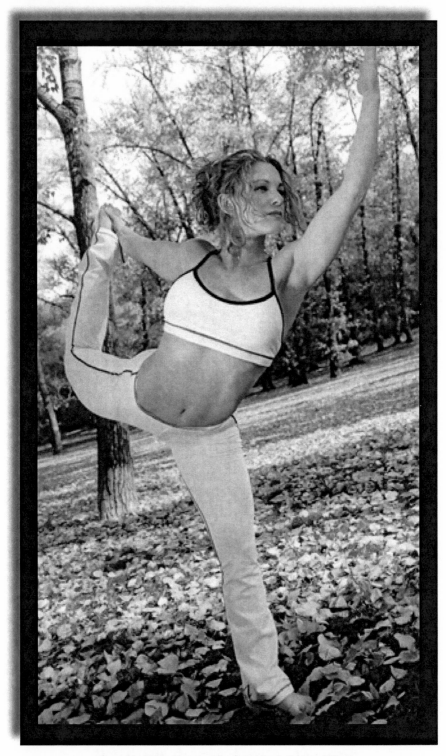

Tanya Lee 2001.  Photographer David Ford.  Calgary, Alberta.

# KEEP IT SIMPLE SUZIE
## laid-back food plan

### 7 step process to get started on these meals

If the theory of athletic nutrition is totally new to you and/or your kitchen has less than 20% of the items on the BodyArt Master Food List, then you have a few more options to pursue before diving into a whole new eating style.

The body works well with gentle progression – keep in mind how when you push a pendulum it will always swing back nearly as hard. The cool thing about being a beginner is that you can start to see changes with baby steps and small adjustments, and you will have lots of room to play with when it comes to the caloric equation.

Below are the BodyArt progressive steps to eating for an active body that have shown sustainable benefits for the vast majority of our students:

1. Eat every three hours.  Perhaps divide your current food intake into 4-6 mini-meals to eat throughout the day.

For example, your current food pattern is likely:
1. breakfast 2. lunch 3. dinner. Go ahead and eat your regular breakfast (1), split your current lunch portion into two meals so you now have early-lunch (2) and late-lunch (3), split your current dinner portion into two meals giving you early-dinner (4) and late-dinner (5).  You just transformed a three meal day into a five meal day.

If you are already eating small meals, but only three a day, then you may want to try adding in one or two small shakes that contain an isolated whey, soy or rice protein and a fruit and/or yogurt/milk.

• eating something every 3 hours
• try some BodyArt meals

**2.** Make this pattern consistent
(give it a month or two)...

**3.** Start to replace your foods with more **quality items** from the BodyArt Master Food List found in this book and the Optimum Body Planner. For example, if you are eating ham and instant potatoes for dinner, change it to lean pork loin and real potatoes. If you are using table salt, switch to unrefined sea salt.

replace high-processed foods with natural choices

**4.** Make this pattern consistent
(give it a month or two)...

**5.** See if you can include a source of **lean protein** (fish, poultry, pork, beef, beans, dairy, powders) and a couple teaspoons of plant oil (olive, flax, canola, coconut, hemp, walnut, etc.) into at least three or four of your meals.

add to your main meals - lean protein and 2 tsp plant oil

*NOTE*
*if you are not training your muscles at least 4 days/week at this point – you may only need to include a protein food source into only two to three of your meals.*

**6.** Make this pattern consistent
(give it a month or two)...

**7.** Examine the types of carbohydrates you are consuming.
A great way to educate yourself is through writing down
all the carbohydrate foods you eat in a day. At the end
of the week, make a list of how many meals you ate with
each of the following: veggies/fruits, grains, sugars. Then
keep making adjustments each week until your ratio of
carbohydrates starts to form a pyramid with veggies/fruits
showing the highest meals and sugars the lowest.

---

• adjust your carbs
• make veggies/fruit out way starch/sugar

---

for example:

week 1: veggies/fruit (1), grains (2), sugars (4)
week 2: veggies/fruit (3), grains (2), sugars (4)
week 3: veggies/fruit (3), grains (2), sugars (2)
week 4: veggies/fruit (4), grains (3), sugars (2)
week 5: veggies/fruit (4), grains (2), sugars (1)

If you want your body sculpting project to be less nerdy, an easier
flow "keep it simple Suzie" style, then I suggest to focus on healthy
portion size and eat four to six of these meals/drinks per day.
Perhaps you'd rather eat until you feel light and satisfied instead of
sticking to the exact weights and portions listed in the meals.

If you want to burn bodyfat and fuel muscles: choose the meals with the "moon icon" for the second half of the day which will increase your veggies, decrease your starch and help to burn more bodyfat as fuel.

If you want to put some muscle size onto your body: eat more meals with the "sun icon" and increase your meals/shakes up to seven per day. If that is too much, try and choose the meals that show the highest calorie count and eat until you are at the higher end of satisfied but do not stuff yourself.

*NOTE*
*Stuffing yourself beyond satisfied can reek havoc on your insides. Let the days go when it was funny to be the human garbage disposal in the platoon.*

If you feel that you are losing energy while you train or if you feel you have a sensitivity to sugars, you may want to try eating mostly the meals listed in the BodyArt Master Food List that feature carbohydrates with a low-to-medium glycemic index. This may help to sustain energy (glycogen) in the muscles for a longer period, and may aid in reducing dramatic water retention and lethargy.

## what if i left my cookbook at home?
If you don't have the cookbook handy or you find yourself on the road and need to prepare a meal, keep the following root guidelines in mind.

The BodyArt Anatomy Of A Meal
* this is based on the quality foods index outlined in the BodyArt Master Food List on page 65.

To reduce bodyfat and maintain muscle:

- 1 protein source
  (meat the size of your palm or a scoop of powder)
- 1/2 starchy carbohydrate (half the size of your fist)
- 2-4 handfuls of fiber veggies
  (a handful is that which fits in your closed hand)
- 2 teaspoons of quality plant oil

To rebuild muscle or if you want to gain weight:
- 1 protein source
  (meat the size of your palm or a scoop of powder)
- 1-2 fist size portions of starchy carbohydrate
- 1-3 handfuls of fiber veggies
- 1 tablespoon of quality plant oil

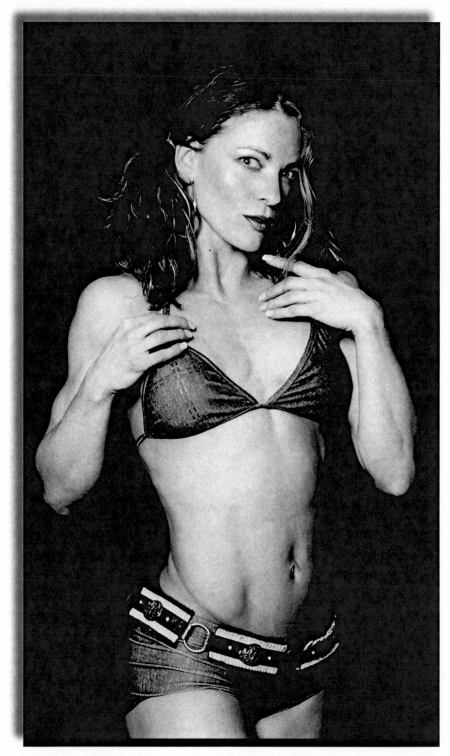

Tanya Lee 2003.   Photographer David Ford.   Lethbridge, Alberta.

# BREAK-IT-DOWN BETTY
## portions/calories

Figuring out the exact amount of food you need to feed your fire is a dynamic equation that can change from meal to meal or week to week depending on various factors including the starting point of your body, what you do for exercise, and the goals you have for your body art project as well as mood which is affected by many factors beyond nutrient depletion to include the brand of medication, herbs, or birth control pill you might use.

Over the years I have heard more comments around calorie confusion than any other topic. Everyone wants to know how much to eat and everybody else has a favorite guru with a theory. Where ever there's frustration and confusion, there will always be people selling quick-fix solutions. There is a lot of information, misinformation, and disinformation about how much to eat for your body goals.

- **when you only count calories, you miss the point**
- **focus on *what* makes up the calories**

If you were to simply eat 1600 calories in random foods off the shelf compared to 1600 calories in BodyArt meals, the numbers would be exactly the same but your body will look and feel much different. In other words, it's not the calories that matter so much but rather what type of food makes up the calories.

In body sculpting and weight management, there are more factors involved than a simple calorie deficit. Generally, an overly simplistic "eat less exercise more" approach may not be the most productive path. When one's focus is solely on calories, they often end up with a lot of empty foods. Many low calorie/fat "tasty treats" (i.e. cereal bars) have been zapped of any remaining nutrients and fortified/enriched with synthetic nutrients, flavors and colors. The thought pattern becomes, "how many cookies, crackers, noodles, hotdogs, chips can I eat for this many calories?".

Even though you lower your calories, your body may not be able to realize that it is bodyfat you aim to lose so the weight you lose may instead come from whatever source it can find. Often, your body is deficient in protein which can signal your insides to turn cannibal and feed on healthy tissues.

Muscle burns calories. When you start to lose muscle, your metabolism suffers so if your goals are to shape your body, lose fat, increase athletic performance, or create more efficient metabolism, focusing just on calories is not likely your best choice.

Many of my clients are amazed when they experience fat loss after I raise their overall calorie intake higher than ever before. The first step in working with your food may not be to lower your calories (even if you want to lose bodyfat), but rather focus on the quality of the calories you are eating.

Not All Calories Are Created Equal

1. Calories (from the Latin root calor meaning "heat") are measured in a lab container (not a human body) recording the heat needed to increase the temperature of 1 gram of water by 1 °C.

2. Most nutrition education teaches that protein and carbohydrates equal four calories per gram and fat equals nine calories per gram. This is an over simplified generalization – not an accurate scientific measurement of food calories. Each food item varies in the amount of calories it has per gram.

If you want to lose 10-30 lbs:
• low calories = temporary loss = 2-4lbs/week
• moderate calories = sustainable loss = 2-4lbs/month

If want to lose more than 30lbs: add 2-3lbs to above

When it comes to managing your body weight, eating a low number of calories will almost always work for short term quick weight loss like bodybuilding competition, making a weight class, or fitting into a wedding dress. Quality calories at moderate number will slow your weight loss down and increase your chances of keeping it off longer.

## a simple formula

Depending on how much bodyfat you currently have and how long you want your fat loss to last, find a calorie range you want to work within and then pick meals from this book that add up to your totals.

For example, you want to lose 15lbs of body fat and you want to keep it off. You decide to focus on 1600 calories of BodyArt meals per day. By the end of one month, check your body weight - if you lost more than 2-4 pounds then add 100 calories - if you lost less than 2-4 pounds, then subtract 100 calories.

*Please Note: Bodybuilders/fitness competitors usually take 8-16 weeks to get super lean, polished and peak their body for the stage. They can lose anywhere between 2-4 lbs/week, but most of them understand that the stage body is not meant to be maintained. They expect and often look forward to gaining weight back after the stage. It's important to understand this for expectation management and prevention of eating/training disorders.*

## you can go on calories alone with the BodyArt meals

There are many theories for what ratios of protein, carb, and fat best work for body sculpting. When your goal is optimum body sculpting and you'd rather not sacrifice your overall health and well-being, there is more to it than fitting into perfectly prescribed numbers. But if you study the range then take the average of what the top professionals are advocating, you may have a better idea of the framework you can play within. I have studied many diets of top athletes and figure models as well as hundreds of my own case studies. From an average of these findings, I came up with the macro nutrient ratios for these meals.

BodyArt meals are one-dish combinations that balance protein, carb, oil, fiber.

When taking a trip, you've got to know your current location before you can map out where you are going next. When it comes to body sculpting, knowing your caloric starting point is the difference between sustainable progression and a body shock that often pushes the pendulum so hard in one direction that it inevitably will swing back with equal momentum/velocity past center in the opposite direction driving you mad.

## find your starting calories

The secret  to working with calories is to figure out your current numbers.  The mistake often happens by "jumping the gun" in a panic to change body shape and then fall prey to a calorie calculating formula that determines what you are "supposed to eat".  Calories may not be accurate so the best way to work with them is as a consistent measurement from where you start to where you are going.

I suggest to start using this book by not using it.  That's right.  First just observe your current habits for seven days without making any changes at all.

Simply observe.  Write down all the details to the following:

> • Everything you put into your mouth (also note restaurant/ pre-packaged foods as they are likely to have more added oils, sugars and salt than those you may make from scratch at home.)
>
> • Everything you do to challenge your muscles (include the type of activity, the intensity you work at and the length of the session)
>
> • Your body weight as soon as you get out of bed, with no clothes on (either before/after emptying your bladder as long as its consistent).

At the end of one week choose three days to average what realistically represents your typical day.  For example, many people start out the week eating healthy, then by Wednesday things start to slip and by Saturday they may be binge eating or in hard core party mode forcing one to feel guilty enough to start the week disciplined.  In this case, a good average of your week could be analyzed by averaging Mon Wed Sat.

Take a rough average of the calories you ate on these three days (add all your calories together and divide by three).  For example: Monday you ate 1600, Wednesday lunch out with the girls took you to

2100 and all the booze on Saturday drove your numbers to 3500.

1600+2100+3500=7200/3=2400.
Your *average* automatic calorie intake is approximately 2400.

Even though this formula has worked for many of my clients, averages are not super accurate representations of your full eating patterns, so remember that this number is loose - not absolute.

example page of the BodyArt Journal Planner

"Pulling averages is like trying to taking a snapshot of someone on a trampoline where a single number rarely can represent the actual full range of dynamic activity. No matter the topic whether its stats/polls/averages related to lifespan or susceptibility to disease given symptoms xyz, rarely can an average/mean ever represent much of anything relevant to everyone equally. It's just a number. 'Quality of life' concepts and even "average lifespan" are really poor statistics with limited relevance." - Wolfgang

---

### treat calorie counting like training wheels

---

## how to know how many calories you are consuming

The calorie amounts in food can be found through many free online calorie calculators, software for your computer, or you can do it the old fashion way and manually calculate with a calorie count book like I and most other competition models I know still do. The BodyArt Journal Planner has a calorie/protein/carbohydrate/fat/fiber chart based on USDA numbers – but only includes the foods you see in the BodyArt Master Food List. Remember to account for sauces/condiments and oils used in cooking preparation. This may be more difficult to measure so my tip is to add about 200 calories to any restaurant meal unless you specifically ask for no oils/sauces added but I would still add 50-100 calories (1 tablespoon of oil is 120 calories).

Once you know how many calories you eat, you may want to start by not changing your calories, but rather exchange the type of food you are eating. If you can sustain 1-2 weeks without changing your calories, but switch from typical North American meals (i.e. macaroni/cheese, pizza, burgers, granola bars, etc) to those in this book, you might well notice a difference.

# 3 body types 3 goals

To fine tune the details of your structured plan, I've outlined a few guidelines that may help according to three different body types and body sculpting goals. There are exceptions to most any rule – so if you get stuck, seek professional guidance that you trust.

## body type #1 EXCESS FAT WITH LITTLE MUSCLE

"I got spare tire no matter what I do: want to firm up."

Does your body look nice/curvy in clothing but for some reason you can pinch way more than an inch, have a spare tire or excess flappy skin that hangs from under your upper arm? This body has little muscle and a high percentage of body fat - a woman may only weigh 110 lbs where 30% of which is bodyfat. Many such women are often trying to change in the gym but rarely see success. If this is you and you are desiring a more toned physique, I have a few suggestions below.

I have seen this scenario over and over among college party girls who tend to go a little too wild with the bottle and the late night drive-throughs that come with it. Over the years metabolism shifts and bodyfat creeps up. My first husband, manager and head bouncer for a nightclub and ultimate fighting promoter would often be asked by the hotties at the club, "What's Tanya's secret to a hard body". He ended up sending all the waitresses and ring card girls to my studio telling them the secret is "80% what you eat" and to "get Tanya's cookbook".

Post-college party girls come into my studio and within months I hear gossip about how "Christy's turning heads in the club – no one knew she was that hot". The secret is small progressive changes to what they are already doing.

FOOD STRATEGY
If you resonate with body/goal #1 listed above, I wouldn't change your current calories at all. I would simply start grazing every couple hours from the BodyArt meals that add up to your current daily calorie intake. The change of macronutrients and food types may be all that is needed, not necessarily a change in calories.

If you want to detail your plan a little more, then choose the meals with the "sun icon" during the first half of the day and immediately after your strength workouts. Choose the meals with the "moon icon" for the second half of the day. This just may increase your potential to fuel your muscles and also burn fat.

EXERCISE STRATEGY
Focus on short, intense strength training sessions – lift whatever weight you can without sacrificing optimum alignment - your bodyweight is often enough. If you want to learn how to move your body safely from your core try my Power Yoga Fusion 8-phase program (bodyartmotion.com) - after you master alignment and gravity, weight training can be so much fun!

If you do cardio, keep it to short sessions of power intervals or low intensity, long duration. Plenty of dance and daily brisk walking may be enough for some to keep it off.

## body type #2  LEAN BUT WANT MORE MUSCLE
"I'm skinny/lean and want more muscle on my frame"

FOOD STRATEGY
In this case I would start the first seven days by adding 200-400 calories to what you are eating now.  Graze on five to seven meals throughout the day and stick mostly to the recipes that have a "sun icon" because they have more starchy carbohydrates.  Discipline yourself to a week at your set calories and if your weight doesn't go up,  then increase by another 200-400 calories.

There's no need to stuff yourself.  If you have raised your calories as high as you can without overeating, then start looking at foods that are calorie dense.  That means foods that pack a high calorie count in a low volume serving.  A handful of nuts can give you 150-300 calories and just one tablespoon of oil is 120 calories.  Also keep in mind that starchy veggies like potatoes usually double or triple the calories of fibrous veggies like broccoli.

It has proven helpful to re-fuel your muscles immediately after a training session with a high calorie drink that contains fast absorbing carbohydrates (glucose/dextrose) and a smaller amount of protein.

EXERCISE STRATEGY
With this goal I also suggest a larger focus on resistance training.  Challenge your muscles to the burn point without sacrificing your body alignment and try to do it in under 10 repetitions of the movement.  For an easy-to-understand book on optimum alignment and core strength, look into my book Alignment Secrets found on www.bodyartmotion.com.


## body type #3  GOT MUSCLE BUT EXCESS FAT TOO
"I'm an athlete got muscle but I'm stalky.  I want more definition."
"I used to have an all-star body. I still got strength but look at me!"

This is the typical scenario of the chick/dude who has muscle who has been athletic or worked out for quite some time (years) yet looks more "stalky" than athletic.  This type often gains muscle rather easily and some women can get frustrated if they enjoy strength training, but see it making their body size larger/stalkier.

FOOD STRATEGY
Where body type #2 might want to eat more calorically dense foods,

you will want to lean more toward "calorically sparse" foods. Fibrous veggies, lean protein, fruit and yogurt could be the staples to your plan. Watch your portion size with starchy carbohydrates, nuts and oil.

If you are eating a lot of junk/fast food or over-processed/packaged food and restaurant food, then I would keep your calories exactly as they are. Plan to graze on 4 to 5 of the BodyArt meals every few hours. Stay disciplined for seven days, keep training and doing cardio, then check the scale. If your diet had a lot of junk in it you may lose 4 to 7 pounds the first week as this is often water loss due to the sudden drop in sodium and preservatives often found in packaged and restaurant foods. After the initial week, if you continue to lose more than 2 lbs/week you could be losing more than just bodyfat, so you may want to increase your calories. If your body weight stays the same for more than 2-3 weeks and you have followed these guidelines eating from these recipes, then you may want to start lowering your calories 100-200 per day and try it for another seven days.

If you have not been disciplined to your eating plan, then I suggest you work on that first before you start changing your calories. Otherwise you can easily create a confusing mess. I wouldn't suggest taking your calories much lower than your body weight with a zero on the end (i.e. 130 lbs. – 1300 calories).

EXERCISE STRATEGY
An increase in cardio and/or training intensity can act as a decrease in calories – but don't go crazy. I have seen many people waste their lives on a treadmill. If your aim is to use stored bodyfat as energy, don't go hard-core on the cardio. If you're gasping for air you are using oxygen for fuel, not bodyfat. If you eat right before you do cardio, you're going to use that food as fuel, not bodyfat. And after you exercise, wait about 20 minutes before you eat and you will give your body more time to use up stored bodyfat.

*If you have done everything listed here and you are still not getting the results you want, then contact an experienced body coach that you trust will respect your values.*

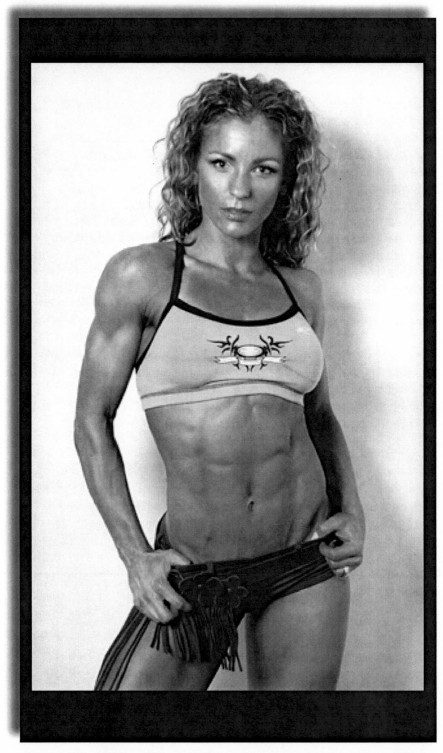

Tanya Lee 2003.  CBBF Figure Nationals.  Back Stage Photo by Doug Schnider.  Edmonton, Alberta.

# CALCULATE IT CATHY
## protein/carbohydrate/fat

When working toward a goal of getting your body fat lower than what is sustainable as in the case with bodybuilding/fitness competition, it is important to know that this can be a potentially dangerous game especially if you are manipulating your sodium/potassium and/or do not have the genetics that the event is modeled after and designed to reward and target. I am not even going to attempt to suggest a plan for event preparation – that would be a whole book in itself. I do suggest hiring a coach that aligns with your ethics and values.

When I was competing as a bodybuilder people used to ask me, "How many hours do you work out in a day to get that lean"? I would tell them it's more about food than training. Bodybuilding is the most nutrition-dependent fitness regime that I have experienced. When you see the big 250 pound guy with 4% body fat, you can almost guarantee that he can tell you exactly how many grams of protein, carbohydrate, and fat he ate that day.

being super lean is more about exact food than training

### revenge of the muscle nerds
To achieve a super hot fitness body, you just may need to be a nerd with a mission! Many champion figure models and bodybuilders have a nerdy side essential to achieving their body goals. Dedication to daily nutrient math is what gives a champ the edge. Macronutrient awareness and carefully crafting six meals a day is a way of life.

Fitness model icon for over a decade and former Ms. Fitness

Olympia, Monica Brant, is known to bring her measuring cups/scales into restaurants. It doesn't surprise me, but nobody outside the fitness arena would call it normal.

Muscle models are ultimately a type of body nerd highly disciplined to tweak the gadgets under the hood to make the machine perform/look awesome while purring like a wild cat. One could also call us artists with an abnormally strong passion/drive/obsession that if we were not able to access the tools to sculpt with we might well go insane. We do it because we must – it's a means to access deeper meaning, freedom, and raw purpose. We shift our values and design our lifestyles around it to achieve it.

So to modify the parental mantra: if you want something bad enough and you are a nerd about it (i.e. "sacrifice social norms") you can achieve it.

## use the recipes as ideas rather than exact meals

If you are a competitor and working with a coach, more than likely, they will prescribe for you a specific amount of calories, protein, carbohydrates and fats that you are to ideally consume in a day. The most effective coaches tend to suggest these ideal numbers along with a list of the types of food they want you to eat and then let you design your own meals.

This allows for more freedom than simply telling you what to eat at every meal which can get really boring and drive someone crazy who enjoys variety. But even if we have the freedom, sometimes we lack creativity which leads many competitors into eating the same thing everyday – boring! – or just downing tuna straight out of the can because at the time you don't feel like thinking about what to do with it. Been there done that. Gets old fast. So I ended up writing the recipes you now have in your hand.

Within the structure of your coaches guidelines you could choose five to seven meals from this book that add up to the numbers that your coach has prescribed – which honestly could drive you batty because it will be really hard to get it exact. Rather, what I recommend is to adjust the recipes to fit your coaches numbers.

For example, say you have already eaten all the fat grams allotted for the day, but the recipe has a teaspoon of oil in it – skip the oil for that meal and continue with the rest of the recipe.

## recreate these meals according to your goals

You can also easily recreate the meals to be individualized for your exact macronutrient ratios needed. Use the recipes as ideas rather than exact meals. If you are competing, chances are that you will have to memorize the grams in your food and will be versed in how to calculate your numbers.

Here's an example on how you may chose to use these meals – say you have planned four of your five meals for the day and what you have left over "to spend" is approximately 32 grams of protein, 32 grams of carbohydrates, and 4 grams of fat. You want to use a can of tuna. Flip open your cookbook to the tuna chapter and find something that looks yummy, take note of the ingredient combination/ meal idea and then recreate the meal according to the measurements of food you need.

BodyArt meals often inspire your own inventions
Have a recipe? e-mail us: info@bodyartmotion.com

Some coaches may specify your carbohydrate numbers into two categories 1. starchy grains/veggies and 2. fibrous veggies. If you need a meal with starches, look for the "sun icon". If you need a meal with no starch and/or fibrous veggies, then look for the "moon icon". Glycemic Index rating of the carbohydrates are listed in the BodyArt Master Food List.

## not competing but want to go all the way?

Q: What if I am not a competitor and don't have a coach, but I want to optimize my training and/or body sculpting project with all the nerdy details?

If your goal is to sustain your fat-burn efforts and fuel your muscle with optimum energy, you may want to take the next step beyond counting calories/portions and enter the realm of macronutrients.

<u>Detail Your Meals</u>
grams of protein
type of carbohydrate
type of oil

## PROTEIN GRAMS

General encyclopedic text provide us these basics. Protein is used for maintaining and repairing muscle, skin, blood, and other tissues. Muscles are built from quality training, not from eating protein. Protein contains nitrogen. When you train your muscles, your body's nitrogen balance often drops. If your nitrogen balance remains in the negative (more nitrogen excreted than consumed) it can present symptoms of a catabolic state when the body's blood and tissues feed on itself. The opposite often occurs when you increase your protein food which results in a positive nitrogen balance – a sign associated with growth and healing (required for training).

On the extreme end, a sustained elevated positive nitrogen balance can indicate signs of kidney damage, as nitrogen is most often measured in urea - a waste product from the digestion of protein which is secreted from the liver and then pulled from the blood by the kidneys.

An equal nitrogen balance may show that your nitrogen intake equals the amount you are releasing and is often associated with a state of muscle maintenance.

I find it helpful to eat for a positive nitrogen balance for approximately six days out of the week, and then have a day or two of "rest" where my protein intake is significantly lower. Next we will focus on designing a start-point structure for how much protein to eat in order to sculpt muscles sustainably.

Assuming you have converted to quality sources of lean meat, egg whites, fish, low-fat dairy, isolated protein powders and/or beans – the next step is to figure out how much protein you need. There are many formulas for protein in the diet, some are designed for short term goals and others aiming at more sustainable programs.

Rancher/farmers must take into account the goals and activity of their horses and vary their protein/nutrients proportionally relative to whether young/rigorous/workhorse/racehorse or need less energy to casually age in the pastures. Too much energy with no place to go is one aspect contributing to fat stores. Athletes and dancers who need to stay lean all year round can eat lower doses of protein than say bodybuilders who often overload on protein to gain as much muscle as possible. Some competition lifters wake in the middle of the night to drink whey protein shakes.

If you have a phobia of "not getting enough protein" or "eating too much protein" and it is stressing you out – there are ways to calm your nerves. There are labs/doctors that offer basic inexpensive metabolic profiles from urine/blood samples. Knowing your nitrogen balance analysis can offer scientific feedback on your protein intake.

A most often recommended easy general formula for daily protein intake for active bodies is 1 gram per pound of body weight. For example a 140lb woman might consume approximately 140g protein/day. If you split 140g evenly across five meals it would come out to about 28g protein/meal. It's not necessary to split it exactly so she can choose to eat 15g at some meals, and 35g at others. This is something that you can play with over time.

The formula above is a mid-range average only and doesn't take into account the intensity or type of training you might do. The more intensely you challenge your muscles, the more protein your body will likely require. A weekend party girl and a dance teacher are going to need different formulas same as a marathon runner is not going to need as much protein as a power lifter. An extreme strength training athlete supplementing with anabolic hormones may be able to use up to 2g/lb, where as the average weekend warrior may only need 0.6g/lb.

>  NOTE: I am stating a truth and neither condoning drug use nor would I bother to take a stance against it since it is a reality that many more are dosing than would admit it regardless of legality or threat of tests that isolate compounds.

**If you want to get more detailed** in your protein calculations, you can look at a different formula that takes into account what your body weight is made up of which is found by testing your bodyfat (BF) to lean body mass (LBM) ratio.

Two women can weigh 140 lbs and have different protein needs. A fitness competitor at 140 lbs and 10% bodyfat is going to have quite a bit more lean body mass to care for than a woman at 140 lbs and 26% bodyfat.

woman #1
(140 lbs x 0.10 = 14 lbs BF) (140 lbs. − 14 lbs BF = 126 lbs LBM)

woman #2
(140 lbs x 0.26 = 36 lbs BF) (140 lbs. − 36 lbs BF = 104 lbs LBM)

So even though both women weigh the same on the scale, one has approximately <u>22 lbs more lean mass</u>, which translates to more muscle.  Chances are woman #1 with more muscle will also have a higher metabolism, so her body could likely process more food than the other 140lb woman.

---

• two women weighing 140lbs can look quite different
• lean body mass is more accurate than body weight

---

This scenario alone seems to warrant the need for a broader set of metrics and formulaic interpretation that includes lean body mass instead of just body weight.  Taking that into account, perhaps 1.2g/lb of LBM could be a better starting point for an active body.

Again, this would have to be adjusted up or down according to the level of training, body progress and/or to address imbalances discovered through blood testing.

Woman #1 who trains intensely six days/week may want to start at 1.3g x 126 lbs. LBM = 164g protein/day, which is roughly 33g/meal.

Woman #2 who trains her muscles 3-4 times/week, may want to start at 1.1g x 104 lbs. LBM = 114g protein/day, which might look like 23g/meal on average.

## TYPE AND PORTION OF OIL

The body sculptor, fighter, dancer or athlete aims to choose their fat source wisely and keep portions to a moderate level.  Too much or too little oil intake may be counterproductive.

Fat nutrients have a lot of punch in a small amount, so the plan is to get the best bang for your buck.  Your body needs high grade quality oil to perform optimally.  Due to commercial ads, more than likely you have heard about good/bad cholesterol and good/bad fats, so let's start here.

Fat from food breaks down into fatty acids many of which can be produced by the inner body chemist while a few others we need to feed our body each day. Food sources breakdown into saturated and unsaturated fats. Most of the fatty acids that we need to eat are found in the unsaturated form of fat which is mostly found in nuts and plant oils. The fatty acids in these oils contribute to vital body functions: heart health, blood pressure, nerve impulses, insulin sensitivity, oxygen transport, and hormonal balance (which signal the body to burn bodyfat).

Unsaturated fat is divided into mono-unsaturated and poly-unsaturated and each of those contain a series of different fatty acids many of which can be supplied by our body processes automatically. The strategy is to keep meat and dairy fats to a minimum while consuming moderate amounts of oils that are loaded with the two main essential polyunsaturated fatty acids that cannot be produced by the body: linoleic (omega-6) and linolenic (omega-3) acids. A 3:1 ratio of omega-6 to omega-3 is said to be the balance required in the human body but due to imbalances that effect the body's fatty acid conversions, an intake of 3:1 ratio may not reflect the same ratio once in the body.

> "We can not we assume that simply ingesting enzyme x or vitamin z in higher amounts is going to have much impact when so many factors on multiple layers are interdependent. If you are low on calcium you cannot just load on calcium. You need to see a calcium/ magnesium/phosphorus triad. Magnesium (Mg) is essential to balancing the effects of calcium (Ca) – for example, Mg gives the tissue elasticity to expand and Ca tension to contract, and with a Mg deficiency Ca can run amok across multiple tissue systems ultimately cannibalizing bone leading to calcification of the soft tissue up in your muscles and/or clogging up the arteries causing higher blood pressure, etc. and still everybody is loading on calcium only to counter osteoporosis (exacerbating bone loss) when 3:1 ratios Mg:Ca (sold only in the UK) are allegedly finding better success for stabilizing the problem.
>
> On a related point, many who push alkaline diets claim the body is suffering from excess acids within and fear

food. The fewest seem to understand how the integrity of a food item changes the minute it begins to combine with the acidic juices of the digestive system. Nearly every fruit (apples to oranges) and many vegetables like tomatoes are as acidic as coffee/coke before they enter your mouth yet end up balancing out most internal systems pushing the pH pendulum back to more alkaline in select tissue systems inside - where it counts. In other words, the lab inside morphs things to the point that what was on the label doesn't reflect what it amounts to inside your body." - Wolfgang

In other words, just eating poly-unsaturated fats at a 3:1 ratio (omega-6 to omega-3) may not be the one-size-fits-all absolute end all answer. The body is infinitely dynamic so there are always various parameters to consider including those yet under-studied, under-documented and unverified.

An athlete or body sculptor may get enough fatty acids with two to four tablespoons of veggie oils per day that could convert to anywhere from 20 to 50 grams per day, depending on your body size. The rest of your daily fat grams are from trace amounts of fat found in the rest of your foods (lean meats, low fat dairy, carbohydrates).

I prefer to mix up the types of veggie oils I use instead of sticking to one. According to Dr. Michael Colgan, author and founder of the Colgan Institute for Nutrition Research, there might be a fatty acid conversion decline after the age of 30 so an athlete of this age group may want to increase and/or lean toward oils higher in omega-3 fatty acids.

Plant and nut oils are delicate, so look for the titles "cold-pressed" and "extra virgin", otherwise the heat processing just may have killed the oil. When cooking, try not to blast the flame or deep fry unless you want to change the chemistry of the oil – which is not likely to your benefit. Different types of veggie oils are also great for topical skin care and massage.

**Approximate unsaturate, monounsaturate, polyunsaturate, omega-6 omega-3 /100 gr of common plant oils.**

| type of oil | saturated | mono unsatu- rated | poly unsatu- rated | omega 6 18:2 (lino- lenic) | omega 3 18:3 (lin- oleic) |
|---|---|---|---|---|---|
| canola oil | 7g | 59g | 29.6g | 20g | 9g |
| coconut oil* | 86.5g | 5.8g | 1.8g | 1.8g | 0g |
| flaxseed oil | 9.4g | 20g | 66g | 12.7g | 53g |
| grapeseed oil | 9.6g | 16g | 70g | 70g | 0.1g |
| hemp oil** | 10.7g | 12g | 75g | 57g | 18g |
| olive oil | 14g | 73g | 11g | 9.7g | 0.8g |
| salmon oil | 20g | 29g | 40g | 1.5g | 1g |
| walnut oil | 9g | 23g | 63g | 53g | 10g |

nutrient facts from USDA government standard

*Coconut oil is scientifically classified as a saturated fat. This category is so far known to increase "bad" cholesterol in those who regularly consume these types of fats. What makes coconut different from most other fats is that is contains medium-chain triglycerides (MCT). MCT oil in it's concentrated form, derived from coconut, has been used by many bodybuilders on low carbohydrate diets as a source of energy. Medium-chain triglycerides have a different, quicker path of absorption and utilization than longer chain fatty acids. MCT's also don't require the typical fat processing through the lymphatic system, but rather shuttle from the liver directly into the mitochondria (the furnace) of a cell to be used as energy which makes it less likely to be stored as bodyfat.*

*For the last two years, I've eaten on average 1-2 tablespoons of virgin coconut oil per day and my cholesterol tested in the normal range. So the choice as to what to believe is yours.*

***Hemp oil contains GLA (Gamma Linolenic Acid) usually only found in evening primrose and borage oil. GLA is an essential omega-6 fatty acid which the body usually produces from omega 3 (linoleic) but may also be required from the diet.*

# TYPE OF CARBOHYDRATE

Many fad diets are advocating no/low carb eating so that the body will use stored bodyfat for fuel. The equation is not that simple.

You can burn bodyfat as fuel without depleting your body of carbohydrate energy. The secret is found in the types of carbohydrates you choose.

The grams of carbohydrates will significantly change within the choice of starch (grains), sugar (fruits), or fibrous vegetables. The BodyArt Master Food List featured in this book and in the <u>BodyArt Journal Planner</u> organize carbohydrates into their respective categories for quick glance reference.

**Fibrous Veggies** are essential roughage that are suggested to be consumed everyday. They will hold the least amount of grams of carbohydrate per portion size. Those looking to control bodyfat may want to further increase these carbohydrates over most starches and sugars – without eliminating any one category.

**Natural Sugars** usually found in fruit and find themselves in the middle between starch and fiber when it comes to amount of grams per portion. Many traditional bodybuilders have a fruit/sugar phobia and will not touch it for four to five months out of the year. Not to say this doesn't work for some people, but the theory is mainly based on the simple/complex carbohydrate model which has been advanced since the introduction of the glycemic index for categorizing carbohydrates.

**Starches** tend to be the heaviest of the three types of carbohydrates with the most grams per portion. Starchy vegetables like potato/yams and grains like rice/oats are often favored by those with super high metabolism, endurance athletes and those looking to gain muscle size. Super high fiber starches like all-bran and lentils are a great addition to control blood sugar and bodyfat.

**Glycemic Index (GI) For Carbohydrates** is based on several factors including blood glucose, insulin secretion, lipoprotein lipase and fat-storage mechanisms, and effects on the pancreas.

The complex/simple model of classifying carbohydrates (starch/sugar/fiber) was more basic where simple carbohydrates like fruit and honey were known to raise blood sugar more quickly than complex carbohydrates like rice and potatoes. In the glycemic system this is not the case. For example a simple carbohydrate like a grapefruit (25 GI) show to have a lower effect on blood sugar than a complex starch like basmati rice (58 GI).

The basic glycemic ratings are simplified for the public to low/med/high (as we have listed in the BodyArt Master Food List), but in more detailed charts are broken down into numbers from approximately 1-100 (based on glucose food source as 100). The glycemic system is much more involved and delicate than the simple/complex model of starch/sugar/fiber. The rating will often change based on what country the food is grown in and what foods the meal is combined with.

For example a russet potato grown in Canada has a rate at 56 GI where the same russet potato grown in USA is rated at 94 GI – that's the difference between a low-to-medium choice and a high-to-higher choice. That same potato will decrease it's GI rating when you add butter or cheese.

Many diabetics are benefiting from the glycemic system of classifying carbohydrates. Athletes consuming a low glycemic diet measured in studies at the Colgan Institute have shown to sustain higher levels of muscle glycogen for longer time periods (translation: their muscles have more energy potential for workouts).

There are also many claims that lower glycemic diets increase fat loss. I tried it out when I was competing and it didn't seem to make a difference for my body at the time. What I may agree with is that a low-to-medium glycemic diet may increase the potential of sustaining fat loss.

Those who train hard and challenge their muscles to fatigue may benefit from consuming a higher glycemic carbohydrate in liquid form immediately after training to replenish the muscle glycogen exhausted during the workout.

There are also several studies indicating the beneficial effects of a low-glycemic diet on certain hormonal imbalances that have been connected to both acne and insulin resistance.

"In a world where 'everything breaks down to theory vs. theory', there is almost always a study to counter another so again, you must be your own best theoretician where your body is your research lab." - Wolfgang

## let's put it all together
### "calculate it cathy" example of protein, carbohyrdate and oil

Cathy weighs 145 lbs and has a bodyfat level of 21%. She trains daily and aims to challenge her muscles during each session. Her workouts include strength training with stability balls, rubber tubing, and weights. Her cardiovascular exercise is about 30 minutes a day, usually some type of dance or jog outside. She tends to gain weight easily and has blood sugar sensitivities.

step 1: find lean body mass
(145 lbs x 0.21 = 30.45 AT) (145 lbs – 30.45 = 114.5 LBM) round to 115 lbs lean body mass.

step 2: exactly how much protein and how do i figure it out?
(115 LBM x 1.3g = 149.5g/day)

or if you don't have the bodyfat measurement
(145 lbs x 1g = 145 g/day)

step 3: what about carbs?
a. post-workout drink
(145 lbs x 0.5g = 73g of high/med glycemic liquid )
b. next meal after drink (73g/2 = 36g)
c. for the rest of the day (73g + 36g = 110g)
d. grand total for the day (73g + 36g + 110g = 219g/day)

step 4: what about oils?
start 11/2  tablespoons of oil/day = 20g
20g + about 3-8g found in whole foods = 23-28g/day

step 5: planning meals
a. totals = 150g protein, 219g carbohydrate, 30g fat
b. post-workout drink = 73g high glycemic carb, 18g whey
c. next meal = 36g carbs, 36g protein, 6g fat
d. rest of meals for the day = 96g protein, 111g carb, 24g fat
e. the approx. schedule for the day may look like this:

|  | food | prot | carb | oil |
|---|---|---|---|---|
| meal 1 | 1 cup extra all-bran<br>1 cup skim milk<br>1 scoop whey protein | 6<br>8<br>24 | 40<br>12<br>3 | 0<br>0.5<br>1 |
| post training drink | (after training session)<br>3.5 scoops of gatorade powder<br>1/2 scoop of whey protein | <br>0<br>12 | <br>75<br>1.5 | <br>1<br>0.5 |
| meal 2 | "No Roll" Chicken Cabbage Roll | 33 | 35 | 4 |
| meal 3 | Mocha Smoothie | 21 | 17 | 2 |
| meal 4 | Creamed Peas (tuna section) | 24 | 24 | 2.5 |
| meal 5 | 1/2 scoop of whey<br>1 tablespoon flaxseed oil<br>1/2 cup nonfat yogurt | 12<br>0<br>5 | 1.5<br>1<br>9 | 0.5<br>13<br>1 |
| totals |  | 145g | 219g | 26g |

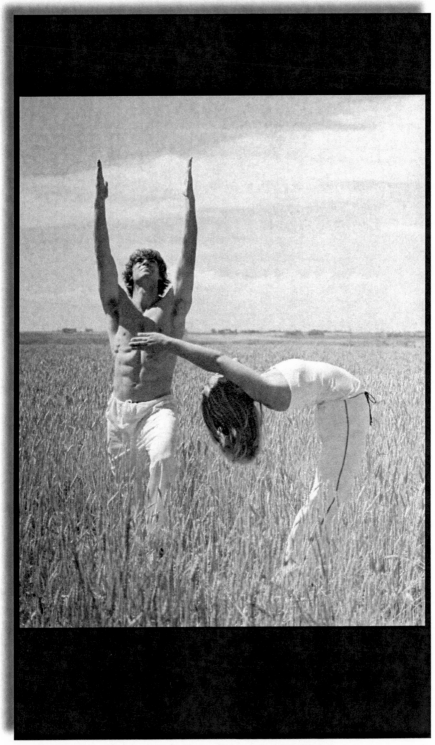

Geordie Day and Brittany Tavernini.  BodyArt Students.

# OTHER HELPFUL TIPS

## plan your meals before your day begins

If you want to stay on track with a detailed nutrition plan, it's helpful to plan out the day's meals the night before or first thing in the morning so that you are prepared to have a smooth flowing day. I know what happens when I skip this step and how radical the difference is when I put this secret in action.

Most mornings, I take five to ten minutes drinking a yerba mate or coffee and plan my meals for the day. Then I prepare most of them, pack up my containers in my tote bag and start my day. It's a great feeling, I don't have to think about 'what to eat' for the rest of the day.

pack a lunch or two! be prepared.

My first husband (a cage fighter) was his biggest and leanest when we lived together. While I was making my meals in the morning, it was just as easy to make his too. So he would go off to the gym for the day with six containers of food. Don't we all just want a private lean body cook!

If you just can't seem to stay disciplined, no matter how much you plan, (say you still end up going to the restaurant even though you packed all your meals) you may want to seek guidance from a seasoned mentor. My 1-on-1 BodyArt Bootcamps focus around the common emotional and mental hurdles as much as on the actual body development process. The inability to stay focused/committed/disciplined can stem from a variety of factors including a lack of essential micronutrients.

## monitor your measurements

To track your body progress goals, it may be effective to focus on your body weight going up or down. I have witnessed beginners keep their weight relatively the same as their bodyfat drops proportionally to muscle gain. The scale alone can be largely deceiving and mostly discouraging if we take it too literally or fixate too much on a direct 1:1 relationship between our progress and scale numbers.

Many of the women whose weight is relatively low but have a large percentage of bodyfat will maintain their weight while sculpting their body. It is not uncommon for a woman to start at 110 lbs with 35% bodyfat and end at 108 lbs and 20% bodyfat.

Most seasoned exercisers who have built a solid muscle base, can usually track progress with a scale. But if you want a more accurate reading, then get your bodyfat percentage taken with calipers by a trainer or health professional you trust. For consistency, it's a good idea to use the same person/method each time.

Consistency is the goal when it comes to measurements. When using a scale, make sure you keep it in on the same spot of the floor, measure yourself at the same time of day (morning is usually most consistent) and don't keep the scale in a place that you have to move it or where it will get kicked around.

**Don't get hung up on the number** – a scale is a measurement tool, not a self-worth gauge. If you have some trauma related to the scale, I understand. But you can trust that there are ways to get around it so that you can use it to help you progress (i.e. don't weight yourself day and night, try once per week or month). Trying to reduce bodyfat without an accurate way to measure can be very frustrating, but with the right context/framing, it can also be done.

the scale is not a self-worth gauge

## "cheat day" craze : moderation is the first thing to go

No, you don't have to be disciplined to your chosen fitness meals all the time. That could drive anyone insane. It nearly happened to me when I spent seven months through two bodybuilding competitions with extreme discipline to every gram of food/drink and every minute of exercise. I did not see the inside of a restaurant or miss one day of training. It took me three years to recover from that experiment.

If you have ever heard of the "cheat day" or "free day" concept it is most likely because Bill Phillips introduced it to the masses. He is one of the more successful business men to turn bodybuilding into a mainstream program. I studied Bill's earlier work before his "Body-For-Life" books were published. Throughout his literature he suggested grazing on a disciplined food plan, similar to the meals in this book, for six days/week and then taking a "cheat day" where one would break from the plan and eat whatever they wanted.

Many trainers today still suggest this routine. While Bill and most trainers suggest you stay in control of your portion sizes - suggesting balance just may be one of those things that is easier said than done.

Over the years I have witnessed many people who could not stop binging on cheat days – to the point that they were making themselves sick and creating self-destructive eating patterns of an "on/off" nature.

Against a wider time frame, I have also seen/experienced this behavior play itself out with some bodybuilding/fitness/figure competitors and professional athletes. In this case the person will devote to extreme discipline for the three to five months of "get lean" event preparation and then cheat season starts the day after the event, eating everything in sight, and often carries on for another seven to nine months until they start the contest phase again. After their career, many of these competitors end up fat and miserable. And the long term physical damage of this type of behavior is surface compared to the deeper psychological torment.

I have my ideas about the psychology behind this type of thing, but that is for another book. Learning to find balance and work past the on/off, good/bad, true/false, black/white mind-trap can be hard work that requires objective awareness development.

Balance is a dance. When it comes to eating, allow yourself some room on the dance floor. Don't over do it, but also don't be lazy.

Rules that are absolute, like "only Saturday can be cheat day" can make someone a compulsive stiff but for others it relieves pressure and they prefer it that way. Keep in mind that a strategy that works for you now, may not be needed in the future and vice versa.

Weekly or bi-weekly cheating on a structured food plan is essential and needs to be practiced for good reason.  If your reason for "why" you are choosing a food is in alignment with your personal integrity, then go for it - just try not to overeat.

Straying from the structure of a body sculpting nutrition plan is about finding what satisfies you most with the least amount of pressure/ worry/guilt.  Play around with it - each person can stray in different amounts and still sustain balance in body-mind-emotion.

"Justification is a bottomless pit of subjectivity"
- Wolfgang

Personal integrity goes hand in hand with trusting yourself. You know what your goals are and with this book you know how to get there.  To take responsibility for your goals is something no one else can offer you and no money can buy.  A plan based on progression allows for healthy cheats.  Body sculpting is a lifetime masterpiece project that never ends, so it's best to choose a path that you can see yourself doing with satisfaction.

---

eat - don't starve.  be kind - don't beat up on yourself.
make sustainable rules - don't parent yourself too harshly.

---

To steadily move forward you may want to remain cheating as much as you already do and each week aim to slightly decrease the daily amount of "cheat" until you get to a point where you can sustain both progression toward your goals and a balanced amount of cheating.

I still use this approach and enjoy both the physical and psychological benefits - body progression while empowering self-confidence.  If your expectations are too restrictive, it will increase the chances of 'falling off the wagon'.  When there's no room for play, each time you have an unplanned 'cheat' it will slowly chisel away at your self trust.

If you go "balls out" on cheat day or cheat season, you may eventually be forced to value balance later when the body begins to show signs of earlier mistreatment.

When there's no room for play, each time you have an unplanned cheat it will slowly chisel away at your self trust.

### decrease worry – it keeps pressure/stress to a minimum

Sometimes we may not have the budget on hand to keep up with the "ideal" daily food intake or we might find ourselves stuck in a situation where the best choices are not available. Letting go of the perceived need for things to be always right, in this case "the right food", may just save you a lot of stress and worry that can eat away at your body-mind-heart.

If you can't get exactly what you feel you need, there is almost always another way to adapt and learn from each situation rather than throwing a temper tantrum or beating up on yourself (i.e. guilt trip self).

Instead of bringing yourself down, look at what you have, assess your options and do the best you can to make the optimum choice and see the opportunity to learn from it. In other words, use what you have to the best of your ability and don't harp on it.

To dance with grace is to keep a flowing rhythm around obstacles, without having to stop and re-start. Know what you value, center in your personal integrity and adjust as needed to sustain progress.

## a few closing notes

Observe, explore and discover what food, cooking, and eating approaches work for your body, values, interests and desires.

When you are ready to sculpt your physical body, rather than going for the quick fix that leads to a bumpy ride, search for a strategy or combination of strategies that complement how you want to live your life.

You don't need to compromise your passions, responsibilities, ethics, values and interests just because you want to eat better and exercise more.

The body sculpting journey will be challenging and you will overcome obstacles, but it does not need to be a cyclical struggle.

Trust what resonates with you. You can listen to the opinions of others and what they believe to be the "right path", but it may be healthiest to understand that you are the only one that knows what feels right for you.

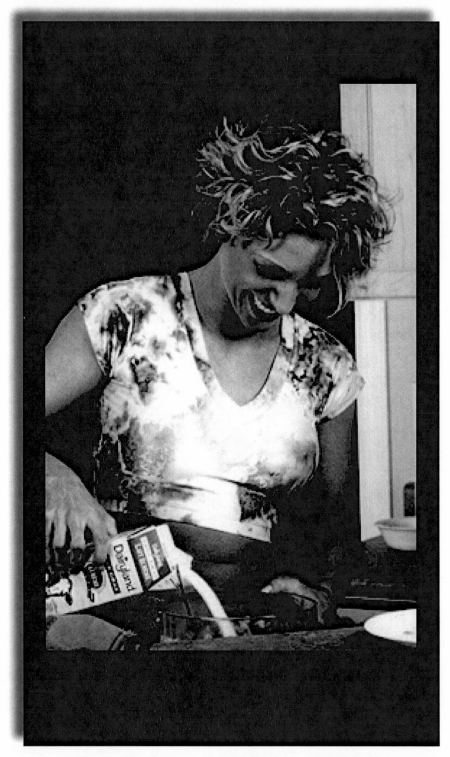

Tanya Lee 2002.  Photographer Terry Goodlad.  Kelowna, British Columbia.

# BODYART COOKING

My kitchen used to be the most boring room in my house. I didn't even consider it a "valid" room. I could never understand why people bothered to decorate kitchens. Well, my kitchen has come a long way since those days. I love my kitchen. I now see it as a sacred space.

Today, my fridge no longer serves solely as condiment storage and the oven is no longer for hiding dirty dishes. I enjoy the time I spend in the kitchen and I know this has an effect on the food I prepare.

As for kitchen organization - forget it!  It is your kitchen and I am not going to tell you how to organize it.  Everyone has a different cooking style.  Everyone has his or her own way of doing anything, which is part of what makes us all unique. You will soon recognize the tools and foods you use most and want to have easy access to.

You will notice that there are no photos of the meals in this book. I have left that part up to what pleases your eye. Sometimes I find it fun and rewarding to create an aesthetically pleasing plate, but that is not the focus of this book.

# conscious cooking

One of the secrets to healthy cooking is in the mindful state of the cook while preparing the ingredients. This theory has been experimented with since the biofeedback experiments of the 1960's and more recently through the work of Japanese scientist Masaru Emoto.

Dr. Emoto's findings show us through imagery how the structure of water molecules are effected depending on the energy state of its surroundings, including thought and emotion.

My first awareness of conscious cooking occurred when one of my friends would make tea. His tea was delicious! When I made the same brand and flavor of tea it just didn't have the same taste. He let me in on his secret. When he made tea he would focus on the person he was making the tea for and think good thoughts about them…wishing them health and happiness. Maybe that's why food never tastes as good as Mom makes it!

When cooking, see if you can clear your mind of worries, clutter and distraction to focus on the ingredients. Bring your attention to the process of preparation and the benefits that will be received from eating the food. Enjoy the textures, colors, and smells of the meal you are preparing.

# time management

One of my goals is to help my clients overcome the barriers of limited time and inconvenience. Most of the meals in this book take between 1-15 minutes from start to finish. If a meal is longer, I have marked them with the clock symbol from the legend.

Do you want maximum results from the information in this cookbook? This approach involves preparing for your recipes ahead of time. Being prepared helps your mind focus on your goals.

How do you incorporate fitness, body transformation, conscious living and still have time to cook and do the rest of the things that keeps your life so busy? This book offers a key. Spend one or two days a week preparing all of your staple ingredients (meats, grains, root vegetables) ahead of time. To some, these meals may be bland - so spice it up at will!

This book also has a "back - up plan" so no worries! If you fall behind on the pre-prep work I have included many meals that require no pre-preparation. After my first long distance tour, I learned how to adapt the BodyArt eating without a kitchen. These "on the road" recipes are also good for when you fall behind on your weekly preparation.

think ahead. be aware. build from a strong foundation.

Having meals prepared ahead of time means less worry about food and more energy for things that are fulfilling. This method will not take over your life. It will enrich your life.

spend 1-2 days/week preparing staple ingredients

# the tools - all you need

You don't really need the big fancy equipment. I spent my first three years bodybuilding with hand-me-down dishes. Actually, my pots were my dad's old camping dishes!

In today's consumer based society, we often have way more than we really need. I can't speak for everyone, but I know that the less clutter I have the less stressful my life becomes.

**MY TOP FOUR PIECES OF COOKING EQUIPMENT**

1. solid sharp knives (small, medium, large)
2. thick wood cutting board
3. solid wood spoon
4. top quality deep-dish stove-top pan

Other than these four, there are some other essentials that may enhance your cooking experience. Keep in mind that we are keeping it simple and basic:

TOOLS THAT MEASURE
A set of measuring cups
A set of measuring spoons
Food Scale (optional)

TOOLS THAT COOK
Rice Steamer
Oven/Stove/Fire
Barbecue

TOOLS THAT MIX
Handheld Potato Masher
Whisk
Traditional Blender
Handheld Blender
Plastic Spatula (pancake flipper)

TOOLS THAT HOLD FOOD WHILE COOKING
  Cookie Sheet
  Pizza Pan
  Big Soup Pot
  Medium Pot (with optional steaming attachment)
  Muffin Tray
  Broiling Rack

TOOLS FOR STORAGE
  "to-go" Containers
  -recycle your cottage cheese & yogurt containers
  -choose material easily broken down by the earth.

OTHER NEAT, HANDY, and OPTIONAL  ITEMS
  Oil Pump (for spraying food)
  Handheld Cheese Grater
  Strainer
  Vegetable Skin Peeler
  Paring knives
  Egg Poacher
  Wide mouth glass jars for spices

## essentials for the table

Taste preferences vary from person to person. The meals in this book are based on macronutrient ratios.  Spice it up as you desire. There are some great "super foods that may add health benefits while also acting as condiments.

These are a few to keep handy on the table:

  - hot sauce (made from cayenne peppers)
  - black pepper
  - unrefined sea salt
    (Redmond Real Salt, Celtic Sea Salt, Himalayan Crystal Salt)
  - liquid amino acids
    (Braggs, Spectrum, etc)

# IMPORTANT!

## FOODS THAT ARE ASSUMED TO BE PRE-COOKED or PREPARED

When the following foods are listed as ingredients in a recipe it is assumed that they are already cooked before hand.

**MEATS**
Chicken Breast, Lean Ground Beef, Lean Cut Steak
(broil, boil, steam, BBQ) *store for max 2-3 days

**ROOT VEGGIES**
Carrot, Potato, Yam, Rutabaga, etc.
(boiled, steamed, baked, mashed)

**GAINS AND LEGUMES**
Rice, Beans, Lentils (boiled, steamed, baked)

**SALAD**
mixture of green and leafy veggies

## pre-cook staple ingredients
It takes only a couple of hours out of the week.  Prepare the above items in bulk quantities.  Store them in containers and stack them in the fridge. Now all you have to do is choose the recipe you want, open the gridge and everything is ready for you! Pick from each of your containers, toss the food combo into your 'to go' container or on the stove in your trusty pan and you're in the game!

From my own experience and validated by hundreds of clients, it takes an average of one or two cooking sessions per week, depending on how many mouths you're feeding.

preparation is worth it - the journey flows more smoothly

# bachelor guide to cooking

CUT OR SLICE   This means to run a knife through something with the purpose of making a smaller version! In this book, there is no difference between chopping, slicing, or cutting. Just get it cut! For the fitness gypsy, use your jack knife and cut your vegetables over your bowl.

CUBE
This means to cut into bite size pieces

DICE
This means to cut very small.

SNIP
This means to use scissors, great time saver and works well with green onion (scallion).

As for the rest of the preparation methods, everything is self-explanatory. Stirring & Mixing are the same things. Blending…yep, use your blender on high. Whip = beat it with a fork or whisk (that metal thing with a lot of wires joined into a tear drop shape). Hint on whipping: the more you whip an egg white, the larger it grows - sometimes 5x size.

*TIP: When handling or preparing food, treat it as a meditation. Imagine whatever you are thinking or feeling is being created as an extra ingredient for the meal. Let go of stress and relax into food preparation. Maybe put on your favorite music and dance some life into your meals.*

# meat | beef poultry fish

## 1. Marinate Meat and/or Salt

First, rub the meat with unprocessed sea salt, then perhaps chose a flavor from the list below - or make your own.

You don't have to marinate, but if you do, you don't have to marinate for long - you can just rub and cook. But, if you let it sit for a couple hours or over night, the flavor will penetrate deeper.

There are many sauces and marinades sold at the grocery store, but more often than not are filled with high ratios of sugar and fat.

Examples of quick, sugar-free marinades you can make yourself:

Lemon Juice & Black Pepper
Lemon Juice & Corriander (great for fish)
Lemon or Lime Juice & Fresh Ginger
Louisiana Hot Sauce
Red Wine Vinegar & Thai Peppers
Balsamic Vinegar & Fresh Garlic
Bragg's Liquid Amino Acids
Tomato Paste & Vinegar with Fresh Basil, Parsley and Garlic

## 2. Massage Meat

Work the raw meat with your hands, just like you would a muscle. Find the knots and press/glide your thumb through them. This step is worth it - makes the meat tender.

### Scale of pressure

Beef needs the most pressure (can be a workout!)
Chicken/Turkey somewhere in the middle
Fish is most delicate

*NOTE if you don't want to get your hands into the spice, you can switch step one and step two.*

# CHICKEN AND TURKEY BREAST

> *NOTE* When you think your chicken is done, cut into it and press down. You want the juices to be clear, not pink. Also, be very careful to clean after you have worked with raw chicken. Salmonella poisoning is not fun!

## boil or poach

Place the chicken breasts in a large fry pan. Cover them with water and turn the heat ½ way between medium and high. Cover with a lid or a round pizza pan. Cook for approximately 25-30 minutes (frozen breasts) or 15-20 (fresh breasts), flipping them around a couple of times. If you cut the chicken into smaller pieces before cooking, the time will decrease. Bored? Add a chunk of fresh garlic or ginger to your water.

## bake or broil

I use this method if I am cooking in the morning. I'll throw the chicken in the oven, go have a shower, get dressed and by the time I'm ready to leave, the chicken is ready to go!

Turn your oven to 375 degrees and place your chicken breasts on broiling rack (a deep dish rectangular pan with a rack set in it). Add a little water in the bottom for easier cleaning afterward. Add optional spices onto the chicken (black pepper, garlic, cayenne, Italian blend, etc.) Cook for 45-60 min. (frozen) or 20-30 min. (fresh), turning them over about ½ way through. I love this method of cooking for fresh chicken breasts still on the bone.

HINT: For the last 5 minutes, turn the heat to broil to make the tops nice and crispy!

## barbecue

Turn your barbecue on to maximum heat and let it get hot for about 5-10 minutes. Once your coals are hot, turn down the flame to medium. Throw your chicken on the grill. Close the lid and cook for 15 minutes. Every 5 minutes flip the chicken over and turn ¼ clockwise.

## GROUND BEEF AND STEAK

### lean ground beef
Cook the beef in a large pot on your stove (option of adding chopped onions). Turn the burner on medium and keep stirring every couple of minutes. Cook until it is no longer pink, which is approximately 15-20 minutes. Then pour the beef into a strainer and allow the grease to drain into a container (so it doesn't clog your sink!). Then place the strainer in the sink and let the water run over the beef while stirring lightly.

### lean steak
Just as in the Chicken directions, you may cook your steak in a pan on the stove, broil it in the oven or outside on the barbecue. The cooking times are about the same of the chicken, but will vary depending on how your like it: rare, medium rare, medium, or well done. You can usually tell how well your steak is done by pressing down with a fork and looking at the color of the juices. Darker red will mean a more rare meat, the more clear the juices the more well done the steak will be.

## WHITE FISH
*Because fish has short cooking times, most of the fish meals can be cooked from raw in the recipes (don't need to be precooked).*

### bake
Preheat the oven to 350°F. Bake for about 12 to 15 minutes depending on the thickness of the fillets.

### steam or poach
Make sure the pan has a well-fitting lid. Fill your pan with enough water to cover half of the fish. Cook on medium heat to bring the water to a gentle simmer. Cover and cook for 4-10 minutes depending on the type and thickness of the fish. Sole takes approximately 4-6 min. while Cod takes about 6-8 min.

# starch | roots and grains

**use a** microwave as an absolute last resort

## ROOT VEGGIES
Potato, carrot, yam, sweet potato, turnip/rutabaga may all be cooked in similar ways.

### boil
With lots of love…Chop your veggie into small to medium cubes and place them in a pot with water (leave enough room for the water to raise when it boils). Turn your burner on high until the water starts to boil, then reduce the heat to medium and allow to cook for approximately 20 minutes for potatoes, other root veggies may take less time.

### steam
I mostly use my rice steamer for carrots and rutabaga / turnip. Chopped the vegetables into bites size pieces and place them in your steamer for about 10-15 minutes

### mash
The recipes in this book will used the mashing technique mostly for potatoes and yams. In preparation for mashing, you may need to cook veggies a little longer so that they are soft.  When you have drained the water after cooking, add a little bit of milk or soy milk and then mash with either a hand masher (old fashion way is always a workout!) or use an electric mixer or hand blender.  Mashed root veggies are wonderful when they are really creamy, so if they look like they are going dry on you, just add a little more milk or water. Sometimes I like to add some low fat sour cream too!

## bake
While bringing your attention to the present moment, gently scrub the skin of the veggie. Pre-heat your oven to 375 degrees.

Wrap your veggie in tin foil with the shiny side facing the vegetable. With a fork or knife, poke the vegetable a couple times on either side. Then place them in the oven on the rack and bake for about 30 - 45 minutes. You will want to turn them over about half way through. Sometimes I like my veggie skins really crispy, so I will unwrap the foil for the last couple minutes of cooking and turn the oven to broil.

## dollar fries
This is mainly for potatoes and  yams. Take a raw potato and slice it into circle disks or into French fry strips. Boil in water for a brief period (5-10 minutes). Then drain the water and toss the potatoes in your favorite spices. With lots of love, arrange the slices on a lightly oiled cookie sheet. Place in the oven on broil for about 5-10 minutes, stirring and flipping about half way through.

## spaghetti squash
I like spaghetti squash because it makes a great fibrous vegetable substitute for pasta spaghetti. To cook this squash, cut it in half lengthwise and place face down in a deep dish with 2 inches of water. Bake at 450 degrees for 30-40 minutes or until the squash can be poked and the fork will easily glide through. Once cooked, scrape out the shells. It should come out like spaghetti strands.

## RICE & LENTILS & QUINOA

### rice
In a pot (for stove use) or in an automatic steamer: measure 1 rice to 1-1.5 water by volume. Cover up and heat till boil. Lower heat and continue to cook till rice is soft and dry. The easiest way to cook rice is in an automatically timed rice cooker/vegetable steamer. Brown rice is higher in fiber so usually takes longer to cook than white rice and may require a 1:2 ratio of rice to water.

### lentils
Lentils need no pre-soaking and cook much more quickly than other dried legumes, but you might want to give them a good rinse before cooking. Place the desired amount into a pot and cover with water. Bring to a boil for 2 to 3 minutes. Reduce heat and simmer until tender. The most common lentils will cook in 10-20 minutes.

### quinoa
Nutty-flavored quinoa is a great alternative to rice. It acts like a grain, but is a seed of a leafy plant. As with lentils, it is wise to rinse the quinoa before cooking. In a pot, measure 1 cup quinoa to 1 1/4-1/2 cup of water. Bring to a boil and then lower heat to simmer and cover the pot. Let simmer for about 15-20 minutes. Gently fluff the cooked quinoa with a fork and let it cool.

## salad | the greener the better

Salad is any blend of raw veggies with a major presence of salad greens. I find it really handy to keep a bin of fresh salad in my fridge. I used to cut fresh greens and combine them to store for use, but lately I have been buying the pre-made bins of organic greens. The life energy stored in salad greens make them one of the greatest foods you can feed your body. Enjoy!

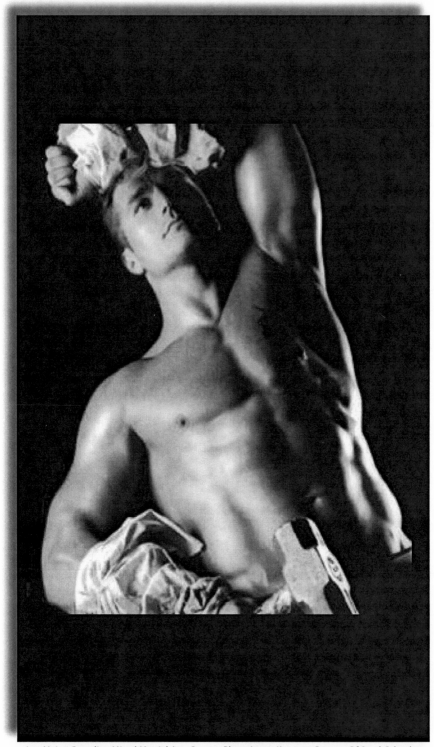

Lee Mein. Canadian Mixed Martial Arts Center. Photo Lorne Kemmet Century Of Steel Calender

# BODYART FOODS

## traditional farming methods

The "organic" label may or may not be the best judge. Whenever I have the opportunity to choose locally grown products, I will support local small business and community farmers - this is the way of life for many communities and families.

When it comes to fruit and veggies, organic labels may be more trust worthy than with other food products, yet there is no way to know for sure. Perhaps the only reason to eat "organic" is if it tastes better to you. Why? Because there may be no way to know for sure whether an item is truly 'organic' or genetically modified.

## animal products

When it comes to meat, eggs and dairy processing practices, it's a 'buyer beware' scenario. Cruelty and overpopulation cause stress and disease which is counterbalanced with amplified nutrient supplements, hormones and antibiotics. I grew up on a cattle farm and was president of my high school 4-H beef club, so I know the value of locally raised meat.

Both my Dads are hunters and fishermen, so I rarely ever ate meat from the grocery store. From a young age, I learned respect for the hunt and often took part helping my dad carry his new kill into the garage where he would then prepare the meat for Mom to cook. Mom grew up in a large family and always made sure every inch of meat was used - nothing wasted.

Not everyone can go out and hunt their own meat or even know of a farmer they can buy eggs and milk from. But for the animals and for your body, every once in a while you may want to check into the origin of the food you chose to eat.

# MASTER FOOD LIST

## PROTEIN

### vegetarian source
1 % Cottage Cheese
Cheddar (low fat)
Milk (non / low fat)
Whey Protein Powder
Yogurt (plain, non / low fat)

### vegan source
Hemp Protein Powder
Rice Protein Powder
Soy Milk (non / low fat)
Soy Protein Powder
Tempeh
Veggie Burgers (Boca brand)

### meat source
Beef - lean cuts
Chicken Breast (Skinless)
Cod
Egg Whites (liquid) 1/2cup =4whites
Egg Whites (powder) 2tsp =4whites
Halibut
Lobster
Mussels
Pork - lean cuts
Scallops
Salmon (canned in water or fresh)
Sardines
Shrimp
Sole
Tuna (canned in water or fresh)
Turkey Breast
Wild Game

## protein powders used in this book (PP)
*you may substitute with your favorite brand*

|  | WHEY | SOY | HEMP | RICE |
|---|---|---|---|---|
| BRAND | pvl<br>natural whey | pro lab<br>pure soy | living harvest<br>pure hemp | rainbow light<br>vanilla |
| SERVING | 31g | 30g | 30g | 27g |
| CALORIES | 120 | 100 | 120 | 100 |
| PROTEIN | 21g | 25g | 14g | 15g |
| CARBS | 5g | 1g | 8g | 7g |
| FIBER | 1g | 2g | 5g | 6g |
| FAT | 1g | 0g | 4g (essentials) | 2g |
| EXTRAS | stevia<br>spirulina<br>lactose free | no sweetners | only ingredient:<br>100% raw<br>organic hemp | spirulina<br>stevia |

# CARBOHYDRATES

## starches
All-Bran *(L)*
Barley *(L)*
Black Beans *(L)*
Bread, multigrain *(M)*
Buckwheat Flour *(L)*
Corn *(L)*
Cornmeal *(M)*
Cream of Wheat *(H)*
Garbanzo Bean *(L)*
Instant Oats *(H)*
Kidney Bean *(L)*
Lentils *(L)*
Oat bran *(L)*
Pita Bread, multigrain*(M)*
Popcorn *(M-H)*
Potato *(H)*
Quinoa *(L)*
Rice, brown *(L-M)*
Rice Cake*(H)*
Rolled Oats *(L-M)*
Shredded Wheat *(M-H)*
Squash Butternut
Sweet Potato *(L-M)*
Toasted Oats *(M)*
Tortilla Wrap *(M)*
Yam *(L)*
Xylitol *(L)*

## simple sugars
Apple *(L)*
Apricot *(L)*
Agave Syrup *(L)*
Banana *(M)*
Banana (over ripe)*(H)*
Blueberries *(L)*
Cherries *(L)*
Date*(H)*
Fig *(M)*
Fructose *(L)*
Glucose *(H)*
Grapefruit *(L)*
Grapes *(L)*
Honey *(L-M)*
Kiwi *(L)*
Mango *(L)*
Maple Syrup *(L)*
Orange *(L)*
Peach*(L)*
Pear *(L)*
Pineapple*(M)*
Raisins*(M)*
Raspberries *(L)*
Strawberries *(L)*
Watermelon *(H)*

## fibrous veggies
Beets*(M-H)*
Bell Peppers (green, red, yellow)
Broccoli *(L)*
Cabbage *(L)*
Carrot *(H)*
Cauliflower *(L)*
Celery *(L)*
Coleslaw Mix, dry *(L)*
Cucumber *(L)*
Green Bean *(L)*
Kale *(L)*
Lettuce (salad greens) *(L)*
Mushroom *(L)*
Onion *(L)*
Pea *(L)*
Pumpkin *(H)*
Romaine Leaves *(L)*
Scallion (long green onion)
Spaghetti Squash
Spinach *(L)*
Tomato *(L)*
Tomato Sauce/Paste *(L)*
Turnip (Rutabaga)*(H)*
Water Chestnut
Zucchini *(L)*

glycemic index rating*
*(H)high [70-100], (M)medium [56-69], (L)low [1-55]*

*based on official tests at University of Sydney. Rates may vary according to country grown, cooking conditions or added foods.

# OILS

If you are cooking with oils, it is best to use low heat, otherwise it may be best to pour oil on the meal after you have cooked it. Plant oils are very delicate.

## liquid

Coconut Oil
Flaxseed Oil (not great for heating)
Grapeseed Oil
Hemp Oil
MCT Oil (Medium Chain Triglycerides) (not great for heating)
Olive Oil
Walnut Oil

## solid

Almonds
Almond Butter
Avocado
Coconut Milk
Ground Flax Seeds (meal)
Hemp Hearts
Peanut Butter (natural - no sugar added)
Pumpkin Seeds
Sunflower Seeds
Tamari (sesame seed paste)
Walnuts

## SPICES
All Spice
Anise
Basil (fresh or dried)
Black Pepper
Cayenne Pepper
Chili Powder
Cilantro
Cinnamon
Coriander
Cumin
Curry
Garlic
Ginger
Onion Powder
Mint
Mustard Powder
Nutmeg
Oregano
Paprika
Parsley
Salt (unrefined sea salt)
Tarragon
Thyme
Tumeric

## CONDIMENTS/MISC
Apple Cider Vinegar (raw)
Balsamic Vinegar
Baking Powder
Baking Soda
Bragg's Liquid Amino Acids
Butter Buds
Cream Cheese (fat free)
Cocoa Powder (unsweetened)
Coffee
Cornstarch
Gelatin
Horseradish
Hot Sauce
Mayo (grapeseed/canola)
Mustard
Nutritional Yeast
Red Wine
Rice Vinegar
Salsa
Sour Cream (low fat)
Soy Sauce (low sodium) or Tamari
Stevia (natural sweetener)
Tea

## EXTRACTS
Almond
Banana
Caramel
Coconut
Lemon
Mint
Maple
Rum
Vanilla

Spices used in meals are optional.
Play and create to your personal tastes.

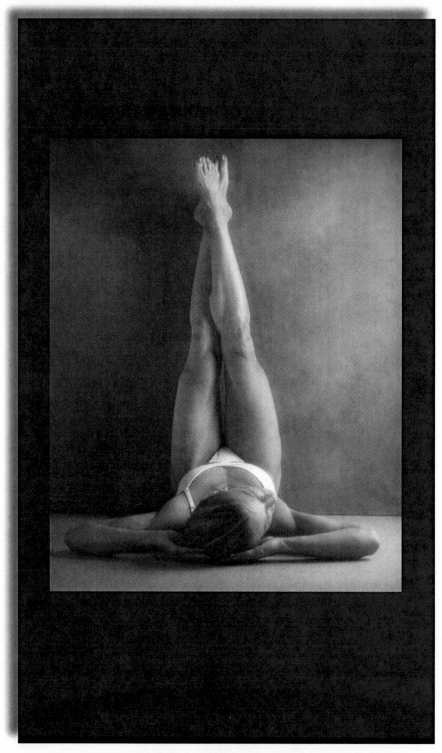

Tanya Lee 2000.   Photographer Lorne Kemmet.   Lethbridge, Alberta.

# SENSUAL EATING

There is much power and sensuality to be felt by focusing a little more intimately on what you are eating and taking into your mouth.

Watch someone eat and you may gain insight into their sensual nature. Do they savor each bite and moan with pleasure providing the cook with feedback?  Or do they watch TV in a recliner with a fork in one hand and the remote control in the other?

The art of optimal food digestion begins with thought, perception and emotion. Then comes the five physical senses of sight, touch, smell, taste, and sound.  Many modern diets have forgotten how important this is becoming numb to one of our most essensual enjoyments.

One of the greatest complaints from dieters is bland food.  Many think they just have to deal with it and force down another can of dry tuna and handful of mini carrots because that's the sacrifice they have to make to eat healthy, clean, right, etc.

Deepening awareness at meal time will bring more flavor and spice without having to load on tones of extra condiments.

Just like paying attention during sensual partner play,  at meal times, one can acquire sensual awareness the more they tune into what stimulates their senses (i.e. spice, flavor, texture, etc).

I took a yoga teacher training course with a monastic woman who spent seven years in eastern ashrams.  During one of our sessions she instructed us to sit in silence during a meal. We were advised to bring all of our focus, attention and thoughts to the food we were eating and to take a full 30 minutes to complete the meal.

With this level of focus many of the students admitted they could actually taste the water and earth that were involved in growing the food.  Some foods like root vegetables tasted more earthy, while juicy fruits provided a more light, watery experience.

Martial artists and yogis have been practicing sense awareness for thousands of years. To these arts, exercising the senses is just as important as exercising the body.

At meal time, breathe, give yourself a moment to center yourself and clear your mind of chatter.  Turn off your cell phones.  Be in the present moment.  Savor the experience.

No need to stop your whole world and bliss out for 30 minutes every time you have a snack, but do try to pay more attention.  Mindless eating is one of the leading causes of overeating.

Often people struggle to kick the habit of smoking because they need the times during the day that they step outside to take a break. The method of grazing every 3 hours may be an opportunity to center yourself throughout the day.

---

no need to bliss out - just try to pay attention.

---

## smell
Smell is one of the most powerful senses for savoring and digestion. When I was a teenager, I loved to sleep in late.  All my mom would have to do to get me out of bed was to cook her famous grand-slam breakfast. The smell would waft into my room and from that point on there was no use fighting it…my feet were patting down the hall!

Note: Animals always smell first to identify whatever is nearby.

## look
Look at your food. Take internal note of what attracts you to your meal. Many of us don't have the time to create an art piece on a plate for every meal. The recipes in this book are stirred together in one bowl, but even with a one-dish meal you can present an array of colors.

In the Eastern chakra theory, the main energy centers in our bodies are associated with different color vibrations, that you can find in most fruits and veggies:

red (foundation and stability), orange (relationships and power) yellow (strength and self-worth) and green (love and balance).

## touch and texture

Touch is another survival sense. When we meet someone we might shake hands or hug depending on where that person is at, or how they blend with our energy. By touching our food, we can also gain a new appreciation for its relationship to our body.

Sometimes I like to eat with my hands (with washed hands of course) - foods like raw spinach, meat, etc. I learned this from one of my yoga teachers. When I eat with my hands I can feel the foods texture before I put it in my mouth. Touch is one of the most intimate senses.

## taste

One would think the sense of taste is always activated while eating, but surprisingly it is rarely developed to its full potential. Usually we are in such a hurry when we eat that taste is more of a familiarity than a true pleasure.

I grew up eating relatively bland foods and never realized it until a gourmet eater pointed it out, so flavor and sensuality is quite relative to ones experience.

## sound

Pleasure can be expressed through sound. Yes, moaning is encouraged during eating! If a meal tastes super yummy, don't you want to express that? It's also great feedback for the cook!

When we chew our food naturally (without talking or listening to another talk), we hear the sound made by the texture of the food and teeth. This can be very satisfying. I enjoy the crisp sound an apple makes when I first bite into it and also the juicy sound it makes as I continue to chew each bite.

Appropriate sound/music can also help create a sensual environment.

# meal legend

| | |
|---|---|
| ☀ | **SUN:** indicates that the meal is higher in starchy carbohydrates or natural sugars.<br><br>Use When You:<br>- finish a good workout (recharge your muscles)<br>- want to build muscle<br>- eat early in the day ( more energy used) |
| ☽ | **MOON:** indicates that the meal often contains less grains, starchy carbohydrates, or simple sugars<br>- more veggies.<br><br>Use When You:<br>- want to decrease extra body fat<br>- want to balance too much blood sugar<br>- eat later in the day (less energy used) |
| 🚗 | **CAR:** indicates that the meal can be made while on the road.<br><br>Use When You:<br>- go on the road<br>- forgot your lunch at home<br>- go camping or backpacking<br>- are on a tight budget |
| 🕒 | **CLOCK:** indicates that the recipe will take longer than 10-15 minutes to prepare or cook. |

PREFERRED SWEETENERS
When recipes call for "preferred sweetener", it's suggesting that you may want to add something sweet to the recipe. If you use the nutrition information provided for each recipe, keep in mind that no calories or carbohydrate grams have been accounted for.

For these recipes non-calorie sweeteners/herbs such as stevia are used as the default. Some people are more sensitive to sugar than others, but I do not recommend using plain white sugar. Small portions of pure maple syrup, honey or raw sugar seem to be better choices. If you are using them in these recipes, please note that it will effect the nutritional information listed, as well as have a blood sugar effect on your body. If your aim is to decrease bodyfat, you may want to keep your sugars to a minimum.

# MAGIC DRINKS
## For the body, mind and soul.

**candied ginger tea**
Soooo good! Slice thin, one large chunk of fresh ginger. Boil it in
about 2 liters of water (depending on how strong you want it. Add
about 10-15 drops of Stevia. Let chill over night. Drink cold or hot.

**comforting chai**
A favorite mountain man classic: from scratch Chai Tea. A friend
made this for me in his VW bus on a cool fall day in the mountains!
In a medium pot on the stove, bring to a boil water and your favorite
whole spices. I like cardamom, anise, vanilla, and a cinnamon stick.
Allow to simmer. Add milk and stevia.

**energizing yerba mate**
If coffee makes your mind too busy, try Yerba Mate - great alternative
to coffee buzz. Rainforest grown and full of antioxidants, Yerba
Mate may stimulate focus and clarity, improve physical energy, aid in
digestion, and support weight loss.

**krakus: the taste of coffee with no caffeine**
Krakus can be found at your local health food store. Krakus has
no caffeine and is an all natural product. It is made from extracts of
roasted barley, rye, chicory, and beet roots.

**master cleanse**
1 quart of Water, 1 Tbsp. lemon or apple cider vinegar, 1/8 tsp
cayenne pepper, 1 Tbsp. honey or maple syrup or molasses.

**sun tea**
Add your favorite herbal, green, or black tea to water. Set it in a clear
glass jug outside with direct contact with the sun for 1-2 days.

**soothing & reviving warm tea**
Look for high quality tea sources at health food stores or local tea
shops. Herbal teas are caffeine free. Green and black teas contain
caffeine unless otherwise stated.

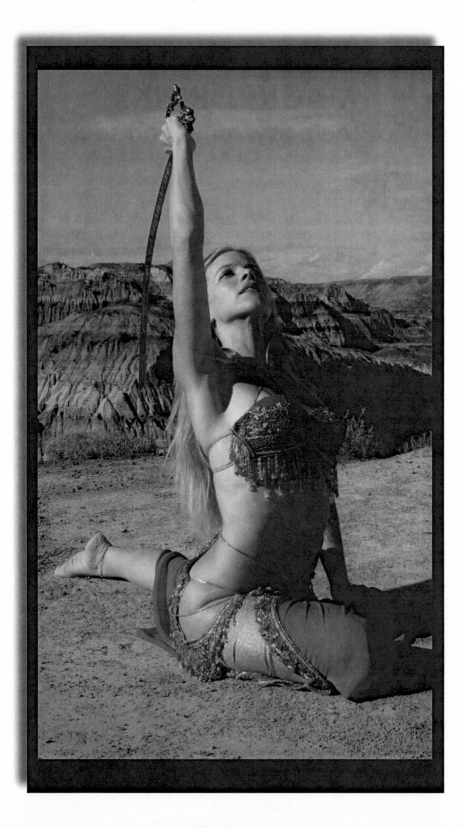

# BodyArtist

## Christy Greene

Professional Dancer and Actor
Owner: Eighth Wonder Productions
www.eighthwonder.ca

Photo by: David Thomas Brown

The body follows the mind and the heart. Doing that which makes us truly happy in spirit, will lead to peace in the mind, success in body and allow us to maximize our creative potential.

Journey journey journey…this is my mantra. I'm learning about baby steps…to slow down in my mad passion for life and learning and to soak up each moment as it happens.

Always a student, I endeavor to discover that which I truly love, and pursue it. I trust my instinct, take risks, and trust the universe ~ what initially appears disastrous is often a gift in disguise.

I have made my passion my work. I perform and teach Belly Dance full time and have found independence in my creativity - and creativity in my independence. I recently combined my two great loves in one stunning project; a Belly Dance Art Film.

# SECTION ONE
# RECIPES

# Vegetarian Meals

plants, dairy & eggs

# MEATLESS MEALS

This section presents alternatives for meat meals. These protein sources are plant or dairy based which are often more easily digestible than meat protein. These are not only great options for vegan and vegetarians, but also for bodybuilders and athletes who require a high level of protein and don't want to eat four to six chicken breasts per day, seven days a week.

A few of the ingredients used in the vegan chapter, you will not see in any other meals. These ingredients are commonly used to balance a vegan lifestyle. Vegan is a style of eating that omits all food from animal sources.

## tempeh (fermented soybeans)
Tempeh has been a favorite food and staple source of protein in Indonesia for several hundred years, but is now rapidly becoming more popular all over the world. It is made by dehulling and cooking organic soy beans which are then mixed with a culture and incubated for fermentation. The culture grows through the beans, binding them into a solid block, which can then be chopped or shaped for use as a protein staple. Tempeh has a firm texture and a nutty mushroom flavor. It is stored and sold fresh, refrigerated, or frozen.

## veggie burgers
Veggie burgers are found in the freezer section of most health food stores. It comes in patty form or ground. Boca is the most popular brand right now and contains 15 grams of protein in each patty. Boca is made from the protein in soy beans and wheat. Boca is often used as a meat substitute with vegan bodybuilders.

## bragg's liquid amino acids
Bragg's liquid amino acid formula is a liquid similar to soy sauce, but surprisingly, is not as high in sodium as actual soy sauce.

## nutritional yeast
Nutritional Yeast is NOT a live yeast. It is a great low sodium bodybuilding food with a complete AA profile, high in B vitamins, and is often used in place of cheese.

One tablespoon of Nutritional Yeast contains
20 cal, 3g protein, 2g carbohydrates, 0g fat, and 1g Fiber.

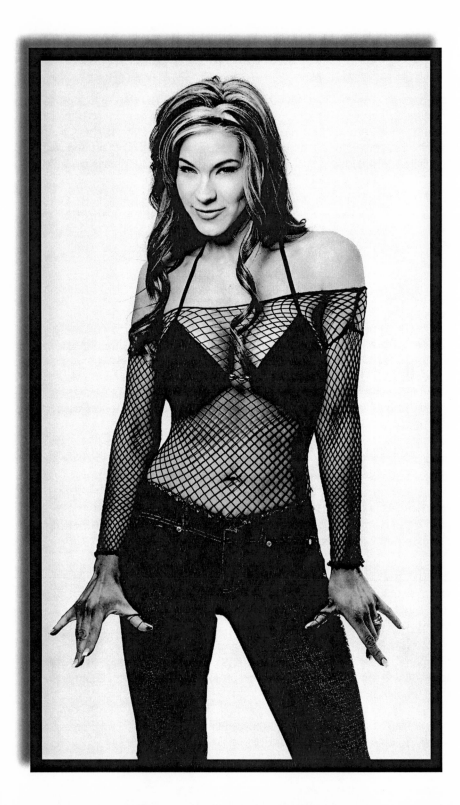

# BodyArtist

## Jacqueline Vos

NPC/CBBF Bikini Competitor
www.jacquelinevos.com

I've always been active and spent much of my life 'performing' in some capacity....however, it was when I started to apply my driven, goal-oriented nature toward taking good care of my body that I really started to see harmony all around.

My primary motivation for eating well comes from within – I noticed huge differences in my general health, and my asthma in particular, as I began to embrace a clean and balanced nutritional strategy. However, the spinoff effects of a clean diet when combined with active living have been a great benefit on the OUTSIDE as well as inside!

I can honestly say that in my early thirties, I now feel younger, healthier and more alive than when I was a teenager. I have so much more energy – and as an athlete, my strength, agility and athleticism have increased immensely. Who can argue with that...?!?!?!

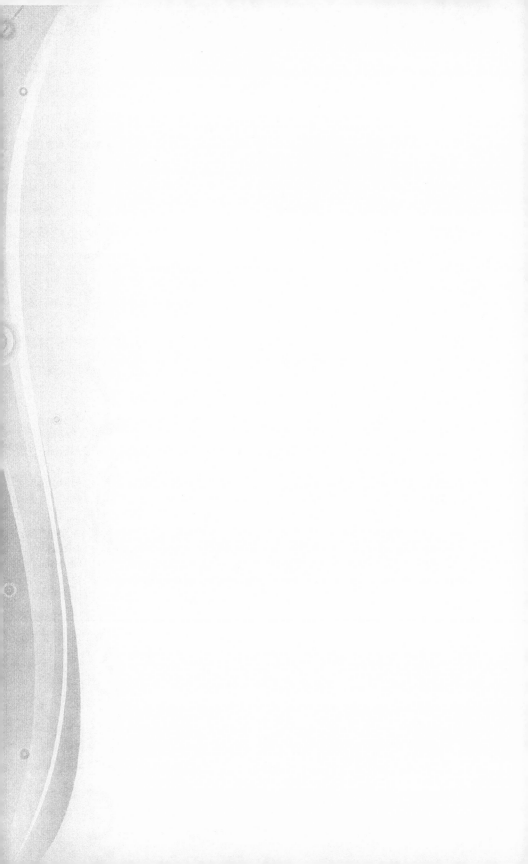

# Special Section
# BIG BODYART COOKIES

## Egg Whites
## Oatmeal
## Protein Powder

These amazing sweet treats can substitute for an entire meal!  You can eat them hot or cold.  They are also easy to throw into zip-lock bags to tote around with you.

**break sweat. don't break stride.**

The idea for Big BodyArt Cookies was inspired by the traditional bodybuilding and fitness model favorite: egg whites and oatmeal.

These BodyArt Cookies have become so popular that a restaurant named 'A Healthy Habit' baked them daily with a new feature flavor each week. Offices ordered them by the dozen to serve at morning meetings.

## homemade meal replacement and energy bars

Store shelves are filled with candy-like options for "on-the go meals". They are often referred to as Protein Bar, Meal Replacement Bar or Energy Bar. The Big BodyArt Cookie is a homemade version made with real food - no preservatives or empty calorie fillers.

### THE ENERGY BAR OR POWER BAR

This cookie will supply you with a greater source of energy. It also includes a good portion of protein keeping your blood sugars in control. These BodyArt Cookies will often include fruit and/or nuts in the recipe.

Use these cookies to refuel and feed your muscles after exercise and see your results enhanced!

### THE MEAL REPLACEMENT BAR

This Cookie is created with a balanced ratio of carbohydrate, fat and protein. It can be eaten as a complete regular meal when you don't have time to cook.

Use these cookies any time of day. If you are looking to decrease bodyfat, use them in the first half of your day or after exercise.

**plan meals. graze often.**

## the egg white

The ultimate real food protein source. When protein sources are compared for complete and easy digestion, and also for their rate of moving into the blood stream (protein efficiency ratio), the egg white rates far above all else. Amino Acids from protein function to build and repair muscles, hormones, antibodies, blood cells, skin, nails, and hair.

## rolled oats (aka uncooked oatmeal)

An inexpensive staple for bodyartists and athletes. One of the highest protein contents of the starchy carbohydrate family, this cholesterol fighting complex carb offers long lasting, stick-to-your-ribs energy.

## protein powder

The original recipe uses isolated soy protein in the base because it is the closest protein powder to act like flour. If you don't want to use soy, then rice or whey protein can be substituted.

Brown rice protein also does a good job acting like a flour, but usually tastes like chalk. Shop around and get a single serving packet to try before you shell out cash for a tin.

If you use isolated whey protein, it will make the cookie drier so you may want to use it in the recipes that call for pumpkin, applesauce or baby food. Also be careful not to overcook the cookie when using whey. But if you do end up with an unbearably dry cookie, just break it into pieces and pour yogurt over it - and it's saved!

substitute soy protein powder for isolated whey
if it ends up dry, put it in a bowl and pour yogurt on it

**break sweat. don't break stride.**

# ✷ BIG BODYART COOKIE

*Servings: 1*
*Per serving: 272 cal, 31g Protein, 31g Carbohydrate, 5.5g Fat, 10g Fiber*

**ADD ½ cup OF FRUIT:**
*322 cal, 31g Protein, 43g Carbohydrate, 5.8g Fat, 11g Fiber*

**ADD 1 TABLESPOON CHOPPED NUTS OR SEEDS:**
*Per serving: 320 cal, 33g Protein, 32g Carbohydrate, 10g Fat, 11g Fiber*

Balance on one foot and stir the following in a big bowl.

   1/2 cup rolled oats
   1/2 scoop (15g) isolated soy protein powder
   1 pinch aluminum free baking powder (optional)
   1 tablespoon flax meal or hemp seeds
   1 dash preferred sweetener
   1 dash cinnamon
   1/4 cup egg beaters (or 2 egg whites)
   1/2 cap vanilla extract

Add water (1/8 -1/4 cup) to make a thick pancake-like batter.

Pour into hot non-stick pan and cook like pancakes, flipping once to brown both sides. You can also bake them in the oven as muffins.

NOTE
Cooks like a big pancake, but looks like big cookie!
Eat hot or take it with you - so handy!

**plan meals. graze often.**

# ☀ BANANA BREAD COOKIE
# (power bar)

*Servings: 1*
*Per serving: 322 cal, 31g Protein, 43g Carbohydrate, 5.8g Fat, 11g Fiber*

Balance on one foot and stir the following in a big bowl.

> 1/2 cup rolled oats
> 1/2 scoop (15g) isolated soy protein powder
> 1 pinch aluminum free baking powder (optional)
> 1 tablespoon flax meal or hemp seeds
> 1 dash preferred sweetener
>
> 1/2 ripe banana (smooshed)
>
> 2 dashes nutmeg
> 1 dash cinnamon
> 1/2 dash ginger
>
> 1/4 cup egg beaters (or 2 egg whites)
> 1 capful vanilla extract

Add WARM water (1/8 cup) to make a thick pancake-like batter.

Pour into hot non-stick pan and cook like pancakes, flipping once to brown both sides. You can also bake them in the oven as muffins.

# ✳ BLACK FOREST COOKIE
## (meal replacement bar)
*Servings: 1*
*Per serving: 319 cal, 33g Protein, 38g Carbohydrate, 8g Fat, 14g Fiber*

Balance on one foot and stir the following in a big bowl.

1/2 cup rolled oats
1/2 scoop (15g) isolated soy protein powder
1 pinch aluminum free baking powder (optional)
1 tablespoon flax meal or hemp seeds
1 dash preferred sweetener

1 tablespoon unsweetened cacao powder
1 tablespoon carob chips
2 teaspoons cherry jello crystals (sugar free)

1/4 cup egg beaters (or 2 egg whites)
1/2 capful vanilla extract

Add water (1/8 -1/4 cup) to make a thick pancake-like batter.

Pour into hot non-stick pan and cook like pancakes, flipping once to brown both sides. You can also bake them in the oven as muffins.

# ☀ BUFFED UP CARROT CAKE COOKIE (power bar)

*Servings: 2*
*Per serving: 248 cal, 20g Protein, 35g Carbohydrate, 5g Fat, 8g Fiber*

Boil the following for a couple minutes until slightly softened.

   2 large carrots (shredded)

Balance on one foot and mix the following in a large bowl.

   1/4 cup egg beaters (2 egg whites)
   1/8 cup buckwheat pancake mix (or ground oats)
   1 scoop (30g) vanilla whey protein powder
   1/2 teaspoon cinnamon
   1 dash cloves
   1 dash nutmeg
   1 tablespoon flax seeds or hemp seeds
   2 teaspoons physillium husk (helps hold it all together)
   2 pinches of preferred sweetener
   1 tablespoon crushed walnuts
   3 figs (diced)

Balance on the other foot and continue to stir - make sure everything is blended well.

Scoop onto medium-heat pan and flatten with back of spoon until they look like little pancakes. Flip half way through.

Or scoop onto a two-side electric grill and close the lid for about 8 minutes.

**break sweat. don't break stride.**

# ☀ CARAMEL APPLE COOKIE
## (power bar)

*Servings: 1*

*Per serving: 335 cal, 31g Protein, 56g Carbohydrate, 5.8g Fat, 11g Fiber*


Balance on one foot and stir the following in a big bowl.

  1/2 cup rolled oats
  1/2 scoop (15g) isolated soy protein powder
  1 pinch aluminum free baking powder (optional)
  1 tablespoon flax meal or hemp seeds
  1 dash preferred sweetener
  2 dashes cinnamon

  1/2 apple (diced small)
  1/4 cup apple sauce
  1/4 cup egg beaters (or 2 egg whites)
  1 capful caramel extract

Add water (1/8 -1/4 cup) to make a thick pancake-like batter.

Pour into hot non-stick pan and cook like pancakes, flipping once to brown both sides. You can also bake them in the oven as muffins.

# ☀ CHOCOLATE BANANA COOKIE (power bar)

Servings: 1

*Per serving: 336 cal, 33g Protein, 47g Carbohydrate, 6.5g Fat, 13g Fiber*

Balance on one foot and stir the following in a big bowl.

   1/2 cup rolled oats
   1/2 scoop (15g) isolated soy protein powder
   1 pinch aluminum free baking powder (optional)
   1 tablespoon flax meal or hemp seeds
   1 dash preferred sweetener

   1 tablespoon unsweetened cacao powder
   1/2 banana (diced small)

   1/4 cup egg beaters (or 2 egg whites)
   1/2 capful vanilla extract

Add water (1/8 -1/4 cup) to make a thick pancake-like batter.

Pour into hot non-stick pan and cook like pancakes, flipping once to brown both sides. You can also bake them in the oven as muffins.

# ☀ CHOCOLATE CAROB CHIP COOKIE
## (meal replacement bar)

*Servings: 1*

*Per serving: 319 cal, 33g Protein, 38g Carbohydrate, 8g Fat, 14g Fiber*

Balance on one foot and stir the following in a big bowl.

    1/2 cup rolled oats
    1/2 scoop (15g) isolated soy protein powder
    1 pinch aluminum free baking powder (optional)
    1 tablespoon flax meal or hemp seeds
    1 dash preferred sweetener

    1 tablespoon unsweetened cacao powder
    1 tablespoon carob chips

    1/4 cup egg beaters (or 2 egg whites)
    1/2 capful vanilla extract

Add water (1/8 -1/4 cup) to make a thick pancake-like batter.

Pour into hot non-stick pan and cook like pancakes, flipping once to brown both sides. You can also bake them in the oven as muffins.

**plan meals. graze often.**

# ☀ CHOCOLATE RAISIN COOKIE
## (power bar)
*Servings: 1*

*Per serving: 364 cal, 34g Protein, 44g Carbohydrate, 8g Fat, 14g Fiber*

Balance on one foot and stir the following in a big bowl.

1/2 cup rolled oats
1/2 scoop (15g) isolated soy protein powder
1 pinch aluminum free baking powder (optional)
1 tablespoon flax meal or hemp seeds
1 dash preferred sweetener

1 tablespoon unsweetened cacao powder
1 tablespoon carob chips
2 tablespoons raisins

1/4 cup egg beaters (or 2 egg whites)
1/2 capful vanilla extract

Add water (1/8 -1/4 cup) to make a thick pancake-like batter.

Pour into hot non-stick pan and cook like pancakes, flipping once to brown both sides. You can also bake them in the oven as muffins.

**break sweat. don't break stride.**

# ✳ CHOCOLATE ZUCCHINI COOKIE
# (meal replacement bar)

*Servings: 1*
*Per serving: 241 cal, 32g Protein, 30g Carbohydrate, 3g Fat, 8g Fiber*

Balance on one foot and mix the following in a bowl.

1/4 cup oat flour or 1/4 cup buckwheat pancake mix
1/2 scoop isolated soy protein powder
1 tablespoon flax or hemp seeds
1/2 teaspoon aluminum free baking powder
1 pinch preferred sweetener
2 teaspoons sugar-free choco jello pudding powder (optional)
2 tablespoons unsweetened cocoa powder

Balance on the other foot and mix the following in another bowl.

1 small-medium zucchini (grated)
1/2 cup egg beaters

Combine the two mixtures together.

Cook like pancakes on your non-stick skillet, or double/triple the recipe and bake in the oven as muffins.

# ☀ GINGERBREAD COOKIE
## (meal replacement bar)

*Servings: 1*
*Per serving: 272 cal, 31g Protein, 31g Carbohydrate, 5.5g Fat, 10g Fiber*

Balance on one foot and stir the following in a big bowl.

> 1/2 cup rolled oats
> 1/2 scoop (15g) isolated soy protein powder
> 1 pinch aluminum free baking powder (optional)
> 1 tablespoon flax meal or hemp seeds
> 1 dash preferred sweetener (try a tsp of dark molasses)
> 1 dash ground cinnamon
> 1 dash ground ginger
> 1/2 dash ground clove
>
> 1/4 cup egg beaters (or 2 egg whites)
> 1/2 capfull rum extract
> 1/2 capful vanilla extract

Add water (1/8 -1/4 cup) to make a thick pancake-like batter.

Pour into hot non-stick pan and cook like pancakes, flipping once to brown both sides. You can also bake them in the oven as muffins.

**break sweat. don't break stride.**

# ☀ KEY LIME COOKIE
## (meal replacement bar)

*Servings: 1*
*Per serving: 319 cal, 33g Protein, 38g Carbohydrate, 8g Fat, 14g Fiber*

Balance on one foot and stir the following in a big bowl.

   1/2 cup rolled oats
   1/2 scoop (15g) isolated soy protein powder
   1 pinch aluminum free baking powder (optional)
   1 tablespoon flax meal or hemp seeds
   1 dash preferred sweetener

   1 tablespoon unsweetened cacao powder
   1 tablespoon carob chips
   2 teaspoons lime jello crystals (sugar free)

   1/4 cup egg beaters (or 2 egg whites)
   1/2 capfu vanilla extract
   1/2 capful coconut extract

Add water (1/8 -1/4 cup) to make a thick pancake-like batter.

Pour into hot non-stick pan and cook like pancakes, flipping once to brown both sides. You can also bake them in the oven as muffins.

# ☀ MAPLE WALNUT COOKIE
## (meal replacement bar)

*Servings: 1*
*Per serving: 320 cal, 33g Protein, 32g Carbohydrate, 10g Fat, 11g Fiber*

Balance on one foot and stir the following in a big bowl.

   1/2 cup rolled oats
   1/2 scoop (15g) isolated soy protein powder
   1 pinch aluminum free baking powder (optional)
   1 tablespoon flax meal or hemp seeds
   1 dash preferred sweetener

   1 dash cinnamon
   1 tablespoon crushed walnuts

   1/4 cup egg beaters (or 2 egg whites)
   1 capful maple extract

Add water (1/8 -1/4 cup) to make a thick pancake-like batter.

Pour into hot non-stick pan and cook like pancakes, flipping once to brown both sides. You can also bake them in the oven as muffins.

# ✳ SKIPPY'S PUMPKIN TREATS
# (power bar)

*Servings: 1*
*Per serving: 323 cal, 37g Protein, 40g Carbohydrate, 4g Fat, 12g Fiber*
*Thanks to Rhonda Lent*


Reciting your favorite poem, stir/whip the following in a bowl.

    1/2 cup of rolled oats
    1/2 scoop isolated soy protein powder
    1 tablespoon flax or hemp seeds
    2 pinches preferred sweetener
    2 dashes cinnamon
    1 pinch allspice
    1/2 teaspoon of aluminum free baking powder
    1/2 cup of canned pure pumpkin
    1/2 cup egg beaters

Cook like a pancake in a low to medium heat non stick pan.
You may want to use a cover to help cook through the pumpkin.

# ☀ ZUCCHINI LEMON CORN CAKES
# (meal replacement bar)

*Servings: 1*

*Per serving:  340 cal, 35.5g Protein, 42g Carbohydrate, 4g Fat, 9g Fiber*

Reciting your favorite poem, whip/stir the following in a bowl.

2 tablespoons of oat flour
2 tablespoons of corn meal
1/2 scoop isolated soy protein powder
1 tablespoon flax seeds
½ teaspoon aluminum free baking powder
1 pinch preferred sweetener
1 cap of lemon extract or lemon jello crystals or real lemon
1 small-medium zucchini (grated)
½ cup egg beaters

Cook it like a pancake in a non stick pan using medium heat.

TIP
To make Oat Flour, grind rolled oats in a coffee grinder or blender on high until they turn fine like flour.

NOTE
Option to substitute oat bran, rice flour, or cream of wheat for the oat flour.

**break sweat. don't break stride.**

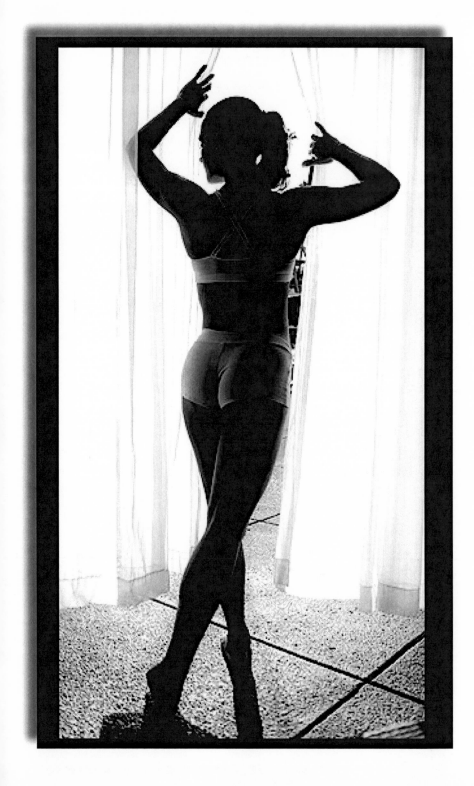

# BodyArtist

## Lea Newman

Officer- US Air Force and Personal Trainer
Ms Fitness USA and Fitness America Competitor

Photo by: Sami Vaskola

I believe that "fitness" is unique to each individual.

For some people fitness is about feeling strong and for other's it's achieving a certain weight loss goal. And yet there are others that are just looking to find the joy of life in exercise and the peace of knowing they are doing something good for themselves.

For me, I am motivated by the desire to inspire, encourage, and motivate others. The best way to do that is to lead by example!

# What to do with:
# DAIRY PRODUCTS

## Cottage Cheese
### (dry curds, non-fat or 1%)

## Cheddar
### (low fat sharp flavor)

## Yogurt
### (plain, non-fat or 1%)

# 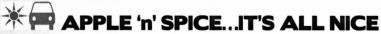 APPLE 'n' SPICE...IT'S ALL NICE

*Servings: 1*
*Per serving: 161 cal, 17g Protein, 18g Carbohydrate, 2g Fat, 2g Fiber*

Seductively swirl the following in your favorite bowl.

    1 cup 1% cottage cheese
    ½ your favorite type of apple (chopped)
    ¼ cup non fat milk
    Pinch of cinnamon (to taste)

For extra sweet tooth: your preferred sweetener to taste

**plan meals. graze often.**

# ☀ CHEESE PIZZA MUSH

*Servings: 1*
*Per serving: 285 cal, 21g Protein, 46g Carbohydrate, 4.3g Fiber, 4.4g Fat*

With care, toss the following in a medium-heat pan.

   ¼ small onion (chopped)
   ½ cup sliced mushrooms
   splash of water

Balance on one foot and stir until softened.
Add the following.

   ½ cup cooked rice
   1/8 cup pineapple chunks or tidbits
   2 tablespoons tomato paste
   3 tablespoons water
   1 pinch basil
   1 pinch oregano
   1 pinch fennel
   1 pinch garlic powder (or fresh garlic)
   ½ cup 1% cottage cheese
   1 tablespoon ricotta cheese

Balance on the other foot and stir until the cottage cheese melts.

# 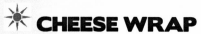 CHEESE WRAP

*Servings: 1*
*Per serving: 345 cal, 26.5g Protein, 38g Carbohydrate, 10g Fat, 8g Fiber*

In a pan, warm up 1 large whole wheat tortilla.

Spread, squirt and sprinkle the following onto the tortilla.

   1 tablespoon fat free cream cheese
   squirt dijion mustard
   pinch of basil

With care, combine the following in a bowl and scoop it down the middle of the tortilla.

   ½ cup 1% cottage cheese
   ¼ med. green bell pepper (diced)
   1 green onion or scallion (chopped)
   1 small handful of baby spinach
   1-2 grape/cherry tomatoes (sliced)

## TORTILLA FOLDING INSTRUCTIONS

step 1:
Fold one end of the tortilla away from you and tuck the edge under the mound of food.

step 2:
Wrap your fingers under the tucked edge and scrape the food toward you using the tucked edge. Firmly pack the food into a log shape that sits in the tortilla fold.

step 3:
Fold in the ends and roll the food-packed log away from you until it is fully wraped in the whole tortilla.

   TIP
   Finish it off in a sandwich grill!

**plan meals. graze often.**

# ☾ CHEESY POPCORN

*Servings: 1*
*Per serving: 295 cal, 14g Protein, 31g Carbohydrate, 13.5g Fat, 6g Fiber*

Air pop 5 cups of popcorn

Spritz on about  2 teaspoons oil

Top with 1/4 cup shredded sharp cheese (low fat)
Shake it around a bit, and you're ready for the movie!

TIP
Also try adding spice like hot sauce or Italian seasoning

# ☾ COLD POWER SOUP

*Servings: 2*
*Per serving: 234 cal, 18g Protein, 21g Carbohydrate, 9g Fat, 4g Fiber*

You're in Spain and a summer breeze blows through your kitchen.
Blend the following on high until smooth.

    1 cup 1% cottage cheese
    1 tablespoon oil of your choice (olive or flax)
    1/8 cup balsamic vinegar
    1/8 cup rice vinegar
    1 green bell pepper (clean out the seeds)
    1 small spanish onion....the purple one! (peeled)
    1-2 cloves of garlic
    1 medium cucumber (chop the ends off)
    1 medium tomato (your favorite kind) or 1 cup grape tomatoes
    juice of one fresh lemon or lime

Keep tasting it and adding ingredients until your taste buds are
satisfied! You may need to add water if you don't use much vinegar.

NOTE
If you save the 2nd portion in the fridge, it tastes even better the next day.  The cottage cheese will separate in the
fridge, so just put it back in the blender for a minute before
you eat.

HINT
Also try this soup with Hemp Protein Powder instead of
Cottage Cheese.

INSPIRATION
A friend from Spain made this recipe on a super hot day in
LA, I had so much energy I had to call it "power soup"!

**plan meals.  graze often.**

# ☾ COLOR THERAPY SALAD

*Servings: 1*
*Per serving: 277 cal, 21g Protein, 37g Carbohydrate, 6.5g Fat, 12g Fiber*

Playfully toss the following in a big bowl.

  1-2 super-size handfuls of fresh salad greens
  1 handful of raw beets (peeled & chopped)
  ½ medium cucumber (chopped)
  1 handful of raw carrot (chopped)
  ½ red bell pepper (sliced)
  ½ yellow bell pepper (sliced)
  ½ orange bell pepper (sliced)
  ½ handful of sprouts
  4 green olives
  ½ handful fresh herbs (I like basil or cilantro)

Balance on one foot and stir the following, then mix it into the rest.

  ¼ cup nonfat plain yogurt
  ½ cup 1% cottage cheese
  1 teaspoon oil of your choice
  spritz of bragg's liquid amino acids
  squeeze of lemon juice

**break sweat. don't break stride.**

# 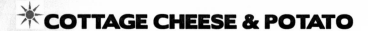 COTTAGE CHEESE & POTATO

## A: Mandi's Baked Potato

Servings: 1
Per serving: 201 cal, 18g Protein, 28g Carbohydrate, 2.2g Fat, 1g Fiber
Thanks to Mandi Parker

Slice the following to create a pocket.

   1 small size baked Potato or yam (3 oz)

Combine the following and stuff it into the potato.

   ½ cup 1% Cottage Cheese
   ¼ cup Cucumber (diced)

## B: Easy Cheesy Potato Mash

Servings: 1
290 cal, 32g Protein, 30g Carbohydrate, 4g Fat, 1g Fiber

With care, toss the following in a medium-heat pan.
Or stir it all into a 'to go' container to heat on the road.

   1 cup 1% cottage cheese
   3oz or ½ cup mash potato or yam (or cubed and boiled soft)
   1 pinch molly mc butter or butter buds
   1 pinch black pepper

   TIP
   If you want a smoother texture, use a hand blender.

**plan meals. graze often.**

# COTTAGE CHEESE TREAT

*Servings: 1*
*Per serving: 270 cal, 28g Protein, 25g Carbohydrate, 6g Fat, 2.7g Fiber*
*Thanks to: Cathy Griffith*

In your favorite bowl or 'to go' container, swirl the following.

¼ cup rolled oats
¾ cup cottage cheese
2 teaspoons fat & sugar free pudding mix
5 almonds
pinch of preferred sweetener

NOTE
You may have to add a few drops of water to moisten (depending on the brand of Cottage Cheese).

TIP
Also try it with brown rice instead of oats!

**break sweat. don't break stride.**

# ◖🚗 COTTAGE CHEESE & YOGURT

*Servings: 1*
*Per serving: 160 cal, 20g Protein, 13g Carbohydrate, 3g Fat, 2g Fiber*

**With Seeds:**
*Per serving: 220 cal, 24g Protein, 14g Carbohydrate, 7.5g Fat, 5g Fiber*

In your favorite bowl or 'to go' container, swirl the following.

½ cup nonfat plain yogurt
½ cup 1% cottage cheese
pinch preferred sweetener to taste (optional)

Optional:
1 tablespoon of hemp or sunflower seeds.

# ( CREAMY CURRY SALAD

*Servings: 1*
*Per serving: 353 cal, 43g Protein, 38g Carbohydrate, 5g Fat, 10.5g Fiber*

With care, blend the following to make a dressing.

1 cup 1% cottage cheese
½ cup nonfat plain yogurt
1 tablespoon oat bran
1 pinch of curry (or to taste)
1-2 handfuls of spinach
1 dash preferred sweetener

Playfully toss the following in a big bowl.

the dressing you just made
2 cups of fresh raw vegetables
(cucumber, mushroom, tomato, brocolli, carrot)
or whatever you have handy.

**break sweat. don't break stride.**

# 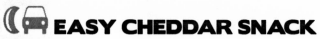 EASY CHEDDAR SNACK

*Servings: 1*
*Per serving: 232 cal, 20g Protein, 18g Carbohydrate, 10.5g Fat, 6g Fiber*

Place two, 1oz slices of low fat cheddar cheese on top of:

6 oz mini carrots
or
1 med. carrot
or
1 med. orange
or
1 sm. apple

**plan meals. graze often.**

# ☀🚘 FITNESS GYPSY CHIPS & DIP

*Servings: 1*
*Per serving: 246 cal, 17g Protein, 21g Carbohydrate, 8.5g Fat, 4g Fiber*

In your favorite bowl or 'to go' container, swirl the following.

   ½ cup 1% cottage cheese
   ¼ cup salsa

Use it to dip the following portion of chips.

   2 handfuls of organic unsalted baked corn/wheat chips

> TIP
> Stir salsa into the cottage cheese, or get creative with spices.

# ☾🚗 FITNESS GYPSY SPINACH CHEESE

*Servings: 1*
*Per serving: 205 cal, 31g Protein, 11.5g Carbohydrate, 4g Fat, 3.5g Fiber*

1 cup 1% cottage cheese
1-2 handfuls of large spinach leaves

With care, walk into the closest grocery store and buy a small container of cottage cheese (make sure you grab a spoon) and some bulk spinach leaves.

Get ready for your picnic! Take a spinach leaf in one hand and scoop a spoonful of cottage cheese into the middle. Fold it over and enjoy!

If you landed in a great organic market you might want to grab some fresh herbs like basil or cilantro to add to the cottage cheese.

NOTE
1 cup of cottage cheese is about ½ of a small container.
If you don't have a refrigerator handy, then buy enough spinach for two snacks that day.

**plan meals. graze often.**

# ( LIME DESSERT AS A MEAL
*Servings: 1*
*Per serving: 240 cal, 21g Protein, 14g Carbohydrate, 11g Fat, 5g Fiber*


With care, mix the following.

> 2 tablespoons ground flax meal
> 1 teaspoon flax oil

Press the mixture into the bottom of a short glass.

In your favorite bowl, swirl the following.

> ½ cup 1% cottage cheese
> ¼ cup non fat plain yogurt
> squeeze fresh lime or lime jello crystals
> pinch of preferred sweetener to taste

Pour into the glass on top of the first mixture.

Eat right away or chill it in the fridge for a while.

# 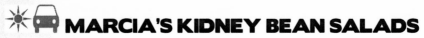 MARCIA'S KIDNEY BEAN SALADS

*Thanks to Marcia Takacs*

## easy option

*Servings: 1*
*Per serving: 290 cal, 37g Protein, 28g Carbohydrate, 4g Fat, 5g Fiber*

In your favorite bowl or 'to go' container, stir the following.

    1 cup 1% cottage cheese
    ½ cup kidney beans (drained and rinsed)
    1 pinch black pepper

Heat or eat cold.

## expanded option

*Servings: 1*
*Per serving: 377 cal, 40g Protein, 40g Carbohydrate, 8g Fat, 7g Fiber*

In a jar, shake the following to make a dressing.
While you're there, shake your hips too!

    2 splashes of rice vinegar
    1 splash of bragg's amino acids
    1 teaspoon oil of your choice
    1 pinch chili powder or cayenne pepper
    1 pinch italian seasoning (low sodium)

Playfully toss the following in a big bowl.

    1 cup 1% cottage cheese
    ½ cup kidney beans (drained and rinsed)
    ¼ cup corn
    ½ tomato (diced)
    1 long green onion or scallion (snipped)
    the dressing you just made.

**plan meals.  graze often.**

# ((🚗 NUTTY CHOCOLATE YOGURT

*Servings: 1*

**WITH COW'S YOGURT:**
*Per serving: 183 cal, 14g Protein, 20g Carbohydrate, 6.5g Fat, 6.5g Fiber*

**WITH SOY YOGURT:**
*Per serving: 197 cal, 15g Protein, 10g Carbohydrate, 11g Fat, 3.6g Fiber*

With a little dance, stir it all together and enjoy the bittersweet bliss of this simple creation!

- 1 cup non fat plain yogurt
- 1 teaspoon of pure cocoa
- 1 pinch of preferred sweetener
- 1 tablespoon hemp hearts (seeds) or sunflower seeds

# ☀ PMS YOGURT

*Servings: 1*
*Per serving: 275 cal, 26g Protein, 33g Carbohydrate, 4.5g Fat, 3.5g Fiber*

Infusing lots of care, into your favorite bowl or 'to go' container, swirl the following.

½ cup nonfat plain yogurt (calcium & live cultures)
¼ cup cooked brown rice (vit. b6)
½ cup 1% cottage cheese (vit. b12 & live cultures)
1 teaspoon cocoa powder (magnesium, iron)
pinch of preferred sweetener to taste

TIP
You can also add a little chocolate pudding powder for an extra sweetness, but I like the bitter-sweet flavor of the pure cocoa with stevia.

NOTE
Adding extra calcium, magnesium and Vitamin B prior to menstruation can help to decrease water retention and irritability. The live cultures found in the dairy products may help keep bacteria balanced.

# ☾ ROMAINE WRAPS

*Servings: 1*
*Per serving: 260 cal, 22g Protein, 17g Carbohydrate, 10.5g Fat, 9g Fiber*

**WITHOUT AVOCADO:**
*Per serving: 168 cal, 21.5g Protein, 13g Carbohydrate, 3g Fat, 5g Fiber*

Wash and separate:

   4 full romaine leafs (boats)

Spread the following over the leaves:

   1 tablespoons fat free cream cheese

Balance on one foot and stir the following in a big bowl.

   ¼ of large or ½ of small avocado (optional)
   ½ cup 1% cottage cheese with your favorite spices
   ½ small zuchinni (diced)
   4 mushrooms (diced)
   cayenne pepper or fav spice

> TIP
> Play with some different veggie combos!

# ✳ SHEPARD'S PIE - VEGETARIAN

*Servings: 1*
*Per serving: 300 cal, 23g Protein, 37g Carbohydrate, 8.5g Fat, 1.5g Fiber*

With care, toss the following in a medium-heat pan.

½ med. or 3oz potato or yam (mashed or baked and smooshed)
½ cup 1% cottage cheese
¼ cup corn
½ green onion (snipped) or dry chives
1 dash cayenne pepper
1 dash paprika
1 dash garlic powder (or real garlic cloves)
1 teaspoon oil

Stir until the smell tantalizes your taste buds.

Serve topped with:
1/8 cup reduced fat cheddar or Nutritional Yeast.

**plan meals. graze often.**

# ((☀ SPINACH DIP

*Servings: 3*

***WITH BAKED CORN CHIPS*** *- 1 lrg handful (approx. 1 cup):*
*Per serving: 294 cal, 23g Protein, 21.5g Carbohydrate, 13g Fat, 9g Fiber*

***WITH RAW VEGGIES*** *- 1 lrg handful (approx. 1 cup+):*
*Per serving: 219 cal, 22g Protein, 13g Carbohydrate, 10g Fat, 7g Fiber*
*Thanks to Michele Theoret*

Raise up onto your toes and mix the following with a blender.

    2 cups 1% cottage cheese
    2 tbsp low fat sour cream
    6 tablespoons light mayo
    2 cups spinach, frozen and thawed
    2 cloves garlic
    1 tsp pepper
    1 tsp dry mustard
    1/8-cup chives
    2 tbsp parsley

# ❨🕐 SUSIE'S COTTAGE CHEESE SALAD

*Servings: 2*
*Per serving: 206 cal, 21g Protein, 13g Carbohydrate, 8g Fat, 2g Fiber*
*Thanks to Susan Murray*

Playfully toss the following in a big bowl and mix well.

    1 tablespoon sundried tomatoes (diced small)
    ¼ cup tablespoon grated sharp cheddar
    1 pinch oregano
    1 pinch fresh basil
    1 pinch garlic powder
    dash of stevia or preferred sweetener
    splash of lemon juice
    2 splashes of rice vinegar

Then stir in the following:

    1 cup 1% cottage cheese
    2 teaspoons oil of your choice
    1 medium cucumber (sliced or chopped)
    1 medium tomato (chopped)

TIP
If you leave it in the fridge for a while the flavors will begin
to dance and explode with more intensity!

**plan meals. graze often.**

# SWEET GREEN BEANS

*Servings: 1*
*Per serving: 257cal, 20g Protein, 40g Carbohydrate, 3g Fat, 7g Fiber*

With care, toss the following in a medium-heat pan.
Or stir it all into a 'to go' container to heat on the road.

2 cups green beans (one small frozen bag)
½ cup basil & oregano tomato sauce (or your preferred flavor)
¼ cup crushed pineapple
½ cup 1% cottage cheese

# ( TAKE IT WITH YOU GREEN BEANS
*Servings: 1*

**WITH HEMP HEARTS**
*Per serving: 266 cal, 23g Protein, 23g Carbohydrate, 10g Fat, 7g Fiber*

**WITHOUT HEMP HEARTS**
*Per serving: 206 cal, 19g Protein, 22g Carbohydrate, 5g Fat, 4g Fiber*

With care, toss the following in a medium-heat pan.
Or stir it all into a 'to go' container to heat on the road.

  ½ cup 1% cottage cheese
  2 cups green beans
  1 tablespoon hemp hearts (seeds)
  1 teaspoon oil

TIP
Also tastes good with a chopped tomato or some salsa!

Or sprinkle flax or sunflower seeds instead of hemp hearts.

NOTE
This is a great no-timer to take with you. The frozen beans
will keep the cottage cheese cool for a couple hours, then
when you are ready to eat, you can have it cold or find
somewhere to warm it up.

**plan meals. graze often.**

# ☾ TURNIP WITH COTTAGE CHEESE

*Servings: 1*
*Per serving: 198 cal, 17g Protein, 20g Carbohydrate, 5g Fat, 6g Fiber*

With care, toss the following in a medium-heat pan.
Or stir it all into a 'to go' container to heat on the road.

    2 cups turnip or 1 large carrot (sliced and lightly cooked)
    ½ cup 1% cottage cheese
    1 teaspoons oil

NOTE
If you have cooked the vegetable prior to making the meal,
then just add care, oil, and cottage cheese. You can eat
cold or heat it up. If you have just finished cooking the
turnip or carrot, then drain the water and stir in the oil and
cottage cheese, so it can melt!

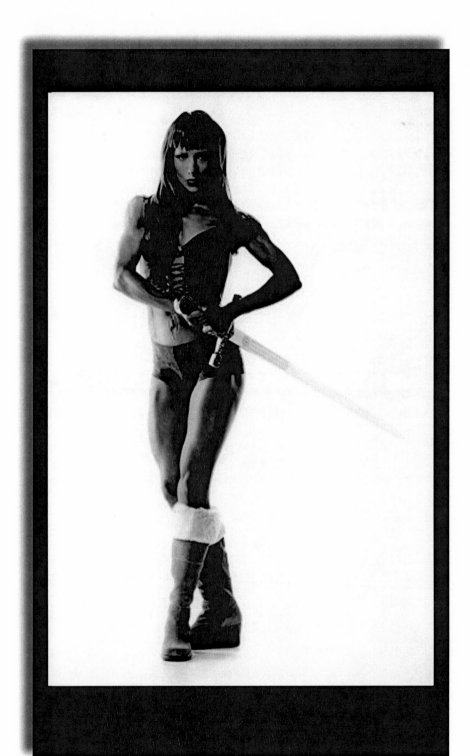

# BodyArtist

## Inga Yandell

ISSA Strength Coach | Performance Nutritionist
Double Impact Fitness | Bare Essentials Magazine
www.bare-essentials.com.au

Photo by: Big Picture Photo

My message to everyone is simple: We need to look within - for it is the courage to take charge of our lives that will transform who we are and where we are at.

The Bare Essentials Magazine is about realizing we are all that is required to make an impact on how we live, what we do and who we B.E.come!

Since 1998, I have be dedicated to providing resources that empower people to live with passion and good health. B.E. "women of action" is a magazine that contains the simplest methods of challenging both mind and body to become strong inside and out. It's dedicated to effective education that supports independence and strength of character.

# What to do with:
# EGG WHITES

## Liquid Egg Beaters
### (whites only)

## Fresh Eggs
### (4 whites = 1/2cup beaters)

## Whole Eggs
### (use yolk + 55cal, 5g fat )

**break sweat. don't break stride.**

#  BIOMAX FRENCH TOAST

*Servings: 1*
*386 cal, 46g Protein, 42g Carbohydrate, 2g Fat, 7g Fiber*
*Thanks to Bob Prosk : Biomax Lethbridge*

Balance on one foot and blend the following.

½ cup egg beaters
1 scoop whey protein powder (vanilla)
¼ cup skim or nonfat soy milk

Pour it into a large plate or deep dish.
Dip both sides of the following into the mixture.

2 slices of sprouted/grainy bread

Cook on medium heat in your non stick pan.
Flip to brown both sides.

> TIP
> Top with 2 tsp of virgin coconut oil (add 60 cal, 7gr fat)
> Top with 2 tsp pure maple syrup (add 25 cal, 7gr carb)

**plan meals. graze often.**

#  BRANDIE'S QUICK BANANA BREAD

*Servings: 1*
*331 cal, 33g Protein, 47g Carbohydrate, 2.5g Fat, 12g Fiber*
*Thanks to Brandie Vander Heide*

With care, blend the following

   1 cup egg beaters
   1/3 cup rolled oats
   1 banana (chopped)
   1 dash of cinnamon

Scramble on medium heat until cooked.

# ☀ BRAVO'S EASY WRAP

Servings: 1
Per serving: 368 cal, 33g Protein, 35g Carbohydrate, 10.5g Fat, 7g Fiber
Thanks to John Rondeau

Stand on one foot and beat the following with a fork or whisk.

1 cup egg beaters
½ cup red, yellow, and green bell peppers (diced)
½ medium tomato (diced)

Warm:
1 large whole wheat tortilla (warm it up a bit)

Spread the following onto the tortilla.

1 tablespoon non-fat mayo

Scoop the egg mixture down the middle of the tortilla.

## TORTILLA FOLDING INSTRUCTIONS

step 1:
Fold one end of the tortilla away from you and tuck the edge under
the mound of food.

step 2:
Wrap your fingers under the tucked edge and scrape the food
toward you using the tucked edge. Firmly pack the food into a log
shape that sits in the tortilla fold.

step 3:
Fold in the ends and roll the food-packed log away from you until it
is fully wraped in the whole tortilla.

TIP
Finish it off with a sandwich grill!

**plan meals. graze often.**

# ☀🕐 CARLY'S FAV BRAN MUFFINS

*Servings: 6 (6 large OR 12 small muffins)*
*Per serving: 195cal, 18g Protein, 32g Carbohydrate, 5g Fat, 19g Fiber*
*Thanks to Carly Broadbent*

Balance on one foot and stir the following in a bowl.

    4 cups of bran or bran cereal
    1 teaspoon of aluminum free baking powder
    ¼ cup hemp hearts (seeds)

Balance on the other foot and stir the following in another bowl.

    2 cups egg beaters
    1 apple (chopped) or ½ cup apple sauce
    4 tablespoons low fat sour cream
    ¼ cup raisins

Combine both bowls.
Pour into non-stick muffin tray
Bake in the oven at 250-325 degrees for 12-17 minutes.

**break sweat. don't break stride.**

# 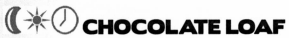CHOCOLATE LOAF

*Servings: 2*
*Per serving: 201cal, 26g Protein, 23g Carbohydrate, 2.5g Fat, 7g Fiber*
*Thanks to: Donna Logue*

Balance on one foot and stir the following in a bowl.

½ cup quick cook oatmeal
1 ½ cups egg whites
1 cup pumpkin
2 packs jello light powder (or gelatin)
8 packs of sugar twin or preferred sweetener
2 heaping t. low fat cocoa
1 tsp extract (banana, coconut, peppermint are good choices)

Spritz the dish of an electric vegtable steamer with nonstick cooking spray.

Pour into the dish and steam for 75 minutes.

**plan meals. graze often.**

# ☀ CHUNKIE POTATO SALAD

*Servings: 1*
*Per serving: 267 cal, 31g Protein, 35g Carbohydrate, 0.7g Fat, 1.5g Fiber*

Scramble:
1 cup egg beaters (add optional butter buds)

Mix the following in a bowl.

  medium size or 4-5 oz potato or yam (boiled, cubed)
  1 long green onion or scallion (chopped)
  1/4 cup non-fat plain yogurt
  1 squirt dijion mustard

Once the eggs have cooled a bit, add them to the bowl.

**break sweat. don't break stride.**

# ☀ CORNMEAL OMLETTE

*Servings: 1*
*Per serving: 266 cal, 30g Protein, 32g Carbohydrate, 2g Fat, 4g Fiber*

Reciting your favorite passion poem, whip the following in a bowl.

  1 cup egg beaters
  1 cup bell peppers, onion, tomato & mushroom (chopped)
  ¼ cup cornmeal
  1 dash basil (fresh is fun!)
  1 dash oregano
  1 dash cayenne pepper

Pour it all into a medium-heat pan and cover it for a minute.

When the top of the omlette becomes white, then FLIP IT. Wait another minute and it should be done!

**plan meals. graze often.**

# 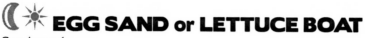 EGG SAND or LETTUCE BOAT

*Servings: 1*

### WITH ROMAINE LEAVES:
*Per serving: 202 cal, 29g Protein, 11g Carbohydrate, 4g Fat, 3g Fiber*

### WITH 2 RICE CAKES OR 1 SLICE SPROUTED BREAD:
*Per serving: 242 cal, 29g Protein, 19g Carbohydrate, 3.5g Fat, 1g Fiber*

### WITH SALAD GREENS AND 1/4 OF LARGE AVOCADO:
*Per serving: 294 cal, 31g Protein, 15g Carbohydrate, 12.5g Fat, 6g Fiber*

### WITH 2 SLICES OF SPROUTED EZEKIEL BREAD & AVOCADO:
*Per serving:454 cal, 39g Protein, 45g Carbohydrate, 13.5g Fat, 12g Fiber*

Reciting your favorite passion poem, whip the following in a bowl.

    1 cup Egg Beaters
    1 dash of Butter Buds
    1 long Green Onion or Scallion
    1 dash Black Pepper

Pour it into a medium-heat pan and cover it for a minute.

    ¼ of a Cucumber (diced)
    1 tablespoon nonfat Mayonnaise
    1 pinch Mustard or Mustard powder

Blend or beat the eggs and the cucumber mix together.
Scoop or spread the mixture on to one of the following.

    2 plain rice cakes
    a bunch of romaine boats/leaves
    1 slice sprouted bread
    big bowl of salad greens and 1/4 avocado
    2 slices of sprouted bread and 1/4 of large avocado

**break sweat. don't break stride.**

# ( FETA SPINACH SCRAMBLE

*Servings: 1*
*Per serving: 185 cal, 26g Protein, 24g Carbohydrate, 4g Fat, 16g Fiber*

With care, toss the following in a medium-heat pan.

 splash of water
 ¼ cup onion (chopped)
 1 clove garlic (sliced)
 handful of button mushrooms (sliced)
 ½ medium zuchinni (chopped small)

Reciting your favorite passion poem, whip the following in a bowl.

 ½ cup egg beaters
 handful of fresh spinach (chopped)
 handful of fresh basil (chopped)
 2 tablespoons feta cheese
 2 tablespoons 1% cottage cheese

Add the mixture to the pan.
Stir frequently, it will be done in just a few minutes.

# ☀ INSTANT FRENCH TOAST IN A BOWL

*Servings: 1*
*Per serving: 306cal, 35g Protein, 29g Carbohydrate, 6g Fat, 6.5g Fiber*

Just after your big morning stretch, toss the following in a medium-heat pan.

   1 cup egg beaters
   ½ cup of dry rolled oats
   pinch of cinnamon
   drop of maple extract
   pinch of preferred sweetener

Stir occasionally.  It should take less than 5 minutes before the eggs are cooked!

Top with:

   1 teaspoon extra virgin coconut oil

> **NOTE**
> If dry, you may need to add a little water for the oats to soak up.

> **TIP**
> If you like, pour a little low sugar syrup or natural maple on top before eating. Adds a few grams of carbohydrate.

**break sweat. don't break stride.**

# ☀ JENNIFER'S BERRY BLAST

*Servings: 1*
*Per serving: 105 cal, 13.5g Protein, 12g Carbohydrate, 0g Fat, 1.5g Fiber*
*Thanks to Jennifer Carter*

Raise up onto your toes, and blend the following.

½ cup egg beaters
1 teaspoon vanilla extract
½ cup frozen or fresh berries
preferred sweetener

With care, pour it in a medium-heat pan and stir like a scramble.

NOTE
Jennifer says, it may look a little different but it tastes great!

HINT
Eat plain or try it with with sugar free (natural) syrup and a slice of rye toast!

**plan meals. graze often.**

# 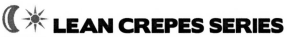 LEAN CREPES SERIES

*Servings: 1*
*Per serving: 100 cal, 15g Protein, 8g Carbohydrate, 0.7g Fat, 1.5g Fiber*

Raise up onto your toes and mix the following with a blender.

- 1/8 cup rolled oats
- 1/2 cup egg beaters
- 1 dash cinnamon
- 1 drop almond extract

Heat a non stick pan to med-high.
Pour the batter into the pan. It will spread thin.
Tip the pan around in a circle so the batter covers the entire pan.

Do a quick dance move until you see your crepe full of bubbles.
Flip it over and cook for a few seconds.

Done!

**break sweat. don't break stride.**

# A: Lemon Cheese Crepes

*Servings: 1*
*Per serving: 150 cal, 23g Protein, 10g Carbohydrate, 1.7g Fat, 1.5g Fiber*

Raise up onto your toes, and blend the following.

  1/8 cup rolled oats
  ½ cup egg beaters
  1 dash cinnamon
  1 drop almond extract

Heat a non stick pan to med-high.
Pour the batter into the pan. It will spread thin.
Tip the pan around in a circle so the batter covers the entire pan.

Do a quick dance move until you see your crepe full of bubbles.
Flip it over and cook for a few seconds.

Make a filling from the combination of the following.

  1/4 cup 1% fat Cottage Cheese
  1 teaspoon lemon rind (thin strips of lemon peel)
   optional sweetener

Scoop it into the crepe and roll for a delicious delight!

NOTE
Option to switch the lemon rind with lemon extract or jello
crystals

# B: Hemp Crepes

*Servings: 1*
*Per serving: 190 cal, 22g Protein, 14g Carbohydrate, 5.5g Fat, 5g Fiber*

Raise up onto your toes, and blend the following.

   1/8 cup rolled oats
   ½ cup egg beaters
   1 dash cinnamon
   1 drop almond extract

Heat a non stick pan to med-high.
Pour the batter into the pan. It will spread thin.
Tip the pan around in a circle so the batter covers the entire pan.

Do a quick dance move until you see your crepe full of bubbles.
Flip it over and cook for a few seconds.

Make a filling from the combination of the following.

   ¼ cup low fat plain yogurt
   1 tablespoon hemp hearts (seeds)

Scoop it into the crepe and roll for a delicious delight!

## C: Maple Flax Crepes

*Servings: 1*
*Per serving: 170 cal, 19g Protein, 15g Carbohydrate, 3.7g Fat, 4g Fiber*

Raise up onto your toes, and blend the following.

    1/8 cup rolled oats
    ½ cup egg beaters
    1 teaspoon flax meal
    1 dash cinnamon
    1 drop almond extract

Heat a non stick pan to med-high.
Pour the batter into the pan. It will spread thin.
Tip the pan around in a circle so the batter covers the entire pan.

Do a quick dance move until you see your crepe full of bubbles.
Flip it over and cook for a few seconds.

Make a filling from the combination of the following.

    ¼ cup nonfat plain yogurt
    couple drops maple extract
    pinch of preferred sweetener

Scoop it into the crepe and roll for a delicious delight!

TIP
Option to switch the maple extract and sweetener for real maple syrup.

**plan meals. graze often.**

# ☀ LITE PANCAKES

*Servings: 1 (about 2-3 large pancakes)*
*Per serving: 303 cal, 31g Protein, 33g Carbohydrate, 6.5g Fat, 9g Fiber*

*WITH 1 TABLESPOON CAROB CHIPS:*
*Per serving: 338 cal, 32g Protein, 37g Carbohydrate, 8g Fat, 11g Fiber*

*WITH ½ CUP CHOPPED FRUIT:*
*Per serving: 343 cal, 31g Protein, 42g Carbohydrate, 7g Fat, 11g Fiber*

Raise up onto your toes, and blend the following.

- ½ cup of rolled oats
- 1 tablespoon flax meal or hemp seeds
- 1 pinch preferred sweetener (optional)
- ¼ cup of lowfat cottage cheese
- ½ teaspoon of aluminum free baking powder
- 1 cap of vanilla extract
- 1 dash cinnamon
- ½ cup egg beaters

Pour onto hot skillet sprayed with non-stick oil spray.
When pancake starts to show bubbles it is time to flip them.

#  MINI PUMPKIN PIES - no crust

*Servings: 2*
*Per serving: 160 cal, 24g Protein, 19g Carbohydrate, 0g Fat, 6g Fiber*

1. Make **Pie Filling** - combine the wet and dry ingredients below.

   ½ cup egg beaters
   ½ cup skim or soy milk
   1½ cups or 1 med can of pure pumpkin

   1/2 scoop (15g) soy protein powder (vanilla or plain)
   2 teaspoons pumpkin pie spice blend, (to taste)
   2 or 3 pinches of preferred sweetener (to taste)

With a ½ cup measuring cup, scoop the mixture (like you would cookies) onto a non stick oven sheet.  Bake for about 30 to 40 minutes at 375 degrees.

> HINT
> If the batter is too runny, add just a little bit of soy powder
> (1 teaspoon at a time…it will thick really easily).

2. Make **Meringue Topping** - You will need a good hand blender or electric mixer. Whip the following until it transforms into a firm white consistency.

   ½ cup egg beaters

Balance on one foot and stir in the following.

   1 cap full of vanilla extract
   1-2 pinches of preferred sweetener (to taste)

After the filling has baked, spoon the meringue mixture onto each one and then broil for a couple minutes until it turns golden color.

> NOTE
> If you want a pie shell, follow the same directions but pour
> the filling into shell instead of scooping like cookies.

**plan meals.  graze often.**

# ☀ EGG & CHEESE SANDWICH

*Servings: 1*
*Per serving: 190 cal, 23.5g Protein, 15g Carbohydrate, 1.5g Fat, 3g Fiber*

Whip the following in a wide base soup bowl and microwave for about 3 minutes.

½ cup egg beaters

Scoop out the egg in one piece.  Place it on top of:

1 slice sprouted/grainy bread (toasted)
1 tablespoon fat free cream cheese

Top with:

1 tablespoon sharp low fat cheddar

# ☾ EGG CANDY - all protein

*Servings: 1*
*Per serving: 63 cal, 13g Protein, 1g Carbohydrate, 0g Fat, 0g Fiber*

Pour the following into a shake container.

 1/2 cup egg beaters

Whip until fluffy white consistency (about 5 straight minutes). I use an old fashion shake mixer or electric hand blender.

Balance on one foot and stir/fold in the following*.

 1-2 drops of caramel extract
 pinch of preferred sweetener

Warm a non-stick pan to medium-heat and scoop the egg mixture into the pan and flatten it out with a spatula, spreading it out to cover the surface of the skillet.

Cover and wait about 5 minutes. The top should be fluffy and solid and the bottom should be lightly browned and easy to remove from the pan.

Eat warm.

 *NOTE
 Play with different flavors of extract and sugar-free powder

  - Cherry extract with tsp of strawberry jello powder
  - Coconut extract with tsp of lime jello powder
  - Vanilla extract with tsp of lemon jello powder

**plan meals.  graze often.**

# ☀ QUINOA HEAVEN (great breakfast)

*Servings: 1*
*Per serving: 341 cal, 33.5g Protein, 34g Carbohydrate, 7g Fat, 4g Fiber*

With care, toss the following in a medium-heat pan.
  1 green onion (snipped into pieces)
  1 handful of mushrooms (sliced/chopped)
  1 teaspoon of oil

Reciting your favorite passion poem, whip the following in a bowl.

  couple drops of maple extract or real maple syurup
  ½ cup cooked quonia (rinse, boil, cover & let sit 15 minutes)
  2 tsp flax meal
  ½ tsp aluminum free baking powder
  dash of corriander
  dash of preferred sweetener
  dash of cayenne pepper

Press it into the pan on top of the mushrooms and onions.
Pour the following ontop.

  1 cup egg beaters (8 egg whites)

Cover and simmer for about 5-7 minutes.
Stir it all together and eat.

TIP
This is one of my most satisfying breakfasts. I'll usually
make up a bunch of quinoa and keep it in the fridge to
have this breakfast for a couple days in a row!

NOTE
I love quinoa (keen-wa). It acts like a grain with a nutty
flavor, but is not a grain. It is the seed of a leafy plant
and is distantly related to spinach. One cup of quinoa is
equivalent to a quart of milk in calcium.

**break sweat. don't break stride.**

# ✳ SWEET MAPLE SCRAMBLE

*Servings: 1*
*Per serving:  324 cal, 37g Protein, 30g Carbohydrate, 8g Fat, 8g Fiber*

Reciting your favorite poem, stir/whip the following in a bowl.

    1 cup egg beaters
    ½ cup cooked brown rice
    2 tablespoons walnuts
    dash of molly mcbutter or butter buds
    1-2 drops of maple extract
    pinch of preferred sweetener

With care, pour into a non stick pan on medium heat.
Stir occasionally until the eggs are cooked.
Should only take a couple minutes.

# ☾ VEGGIE OMLETTE

*Servings: 1*
*Per serving:  239 cal, 35g Protein, 16g Carbohydrate, 3.4g Fat, 5g Fiber*

Reciting your favorite poem, whip/stir the following in a bowl.

    1 cup egg beaters
    1 tablespoon raw pumpkin seeds
    dash of molly mcbutter or butter buds
    ½ small onion (chopped)
    handful of button mushrooms (sliced)
    1 cup brocolli (chopped small)
    ½ cup green and red bell peppers (chopped)

Pour into a medium-heated non-stick pan.
Watch the pan until the top of the omlette turns whiteish.
See if you can flip the whole thing over in one piece!

If managed to flip the omlette in one piece, then make a line down
the center of the egg with:

    2 tablespoons nonfat cottage cheese

Fold both ends of the omlette over top the cheese line down the
center. Cover and let the cheese melt.

If the omlette broke apart when you flipped it, then just add the
cottage cheese and stir everything around like scrambled eggs.
Either way, its all fun!

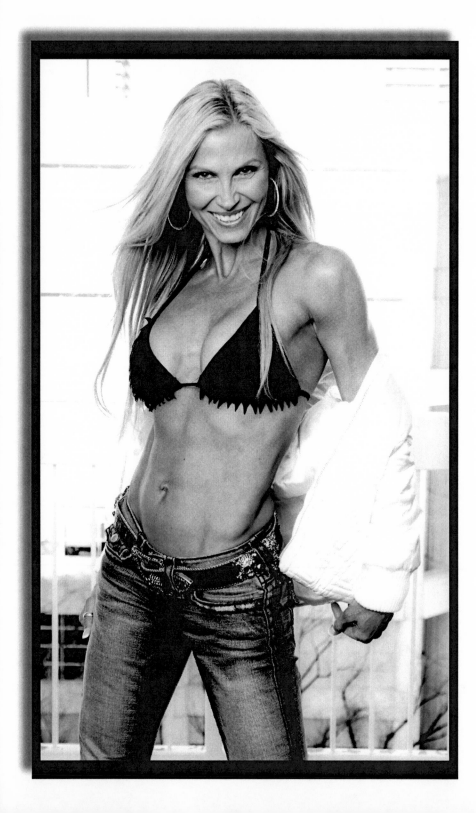

# BodyArtist

## Shauna Sky Romano

Former World Champion in the Sport of Skeleton
Fitness Model Competitor | Kiniesiologist
Owner: Love2Move High Performance Coaching
www.shaunasky.com

I am honored to say that this is my life and I am "living the dream!"

I love to share my knowledge of training and high performance. My passion comes from working with people to find and connect with the profound wisdom that our physical bodies manifest. Altering perceptions, creating vision and inspiring others to take their health, wellness, and whatever idea they have of fitness to whatever level is right for them.

I am inspired and driven by my love of movement and the deep respect I have for the human body. I had my pelvic floor completely re-built after the birth of my son and the journey back to health has been empowering. My 2 children Alexa and Mateo have been my greatest teachers.

I've learnt that we are all the same....that to find our deepest compassion and empathy is truly to find peace. Be true to yourself. Listen deeply. Look up and look in....

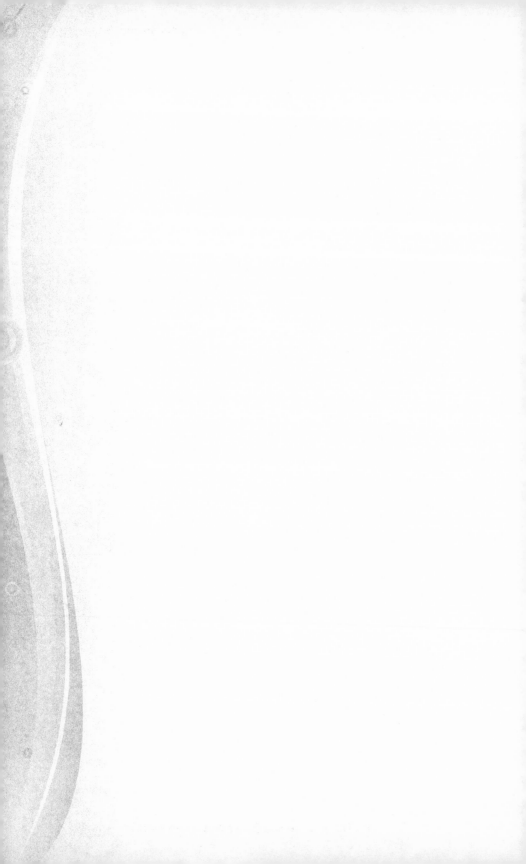

# What to do with:
# PROTEIN POWDERS

## Whey
(isolate)

## Soy
(isolate)

## Hemp
(raw)

## Rice
(just the protein, not the carb parts)

**break sweat. don't break stride.**

## Why protein powder?

Powder protein is affordable and gives your body a break from the overload of meat digestion.

Protein powders are also:
- easy for travel
- need no refrigeration
- quick for snacks and when you're not prepared
- full of flavor variety

There is an array of different protein foods in powder form such as whey, soy, rice, hemp, and egg. There also are numerous flavors and brands.

As far as the body's "return on investment" is concerned, athletes over decades have agreed that whey and egg are the King and Queen of protein.

WHEY: When shopping for whey protein powder look for "isolated protein". If it only says "concentrated protein" that means it has lower protein content and compensates with more fat, cholesterol, and lactose.

SOY: Look for "isolated soy", Supro Brandâ seems to be a reputable name. Look at the carbohydrate grams, if it's more than 5 grams per 30 gram serving you are getting more ingredients than just isolated soy protein.

HEMP: An ancient food, but relatively new to our markets. It does taste a little "greener" than the others.  Hemp protein usually comes in 100% pure raw hemp protein with no other ingredients. This protein is usually accompanied with extra fiber and essential fatty acids.

RICE: Rice is a starchy grain, but in this product protein is removed from the rice and changed to powder.  I tried several rice protien powders - many of them taste like chalk. Try a few out.

Refer to the ingredients chapter for the macronutrient breakdown of the powders used in these recipes

**plan meals.  graze often.**

# ☀ AFTER EIGHT SMOOTHIE
*Servings: 1*

**WITH WHEY PROTEIN & COW'S MILK:**
*Per serving: 317 cal, 33g Protein, 40g Carbohydrate, 5g Fat, 8gFiber*

**WITH RICE PROTEIN & SOY MILK:**
*Per serving: 281 cal, 25g Protein, 40g Carbohydrate, 6g Fat, 14gFiber*

**WITH HEMP PROTEIN & SOY MILK:**
*Per serving: 301 cal, 24g Protein, 41g Carbohydrate, 8g Fat, 14gFiber*

Raise up onto your toes and mix the following with a blender.

- 1 scoop chocolate or vanilla protein powder
- ½ frozen banana
- 1 cup non fat milk or soy milk
- handful of fresh mint leaves (or use mint extract)
- 2 tablespoons of carob powder or unsweetened cocoa powder

- 1 tablespoon of unsweetened carob chips

NOTE
Add the carob chips before or after you blend.

**break sweat. don't break stride.**

#  CAROB DATE SMOOTHIE

*Servings: 1*
*thanks to Kelly Phipps*

### WITH WHEY PROTEIN & COW'S MILK:
*Per serving: 408 cal, 34g Protein, 58g Carbohydrate, 8.5g Fat, 8g Fiber*

### WITH RICE PROTEIN & SOY MILK:
*Per serving: 372 cal, 26g Protein, 58g Carbohydrate, 9g Fat, 14g Fiber*

### WITH HEMP PROTEIN & SOY MILK:
*Per serving: 392 cal, 25g Protein, 59g Carbohydrate, 11g Fat, 14g Fiber*

Raise up onto your toes and mix the following with a blender.

   1 scoop chocolate or vanilla protein powder
   ½ frozen banana
   1 cup non fat milk or soy milk
   1 tablespoon sunflower seeds
   2 pitted dates
   2 tablespoons of carob powder or unsweetened cocoa powder

TIP
"the trick to a good smoothie is the frozen bananas.
Cut them into slices and store them in the freezer."

HINT
Because of the high glycemic rating of the dates, this
smooth could be a great candidate for a post-training
muscle refresher.

**plan meals. graze often.**

# ☾ CARROT & RAISIN SALAD

*Servings: 1*
*Per serving: 238cal, 22g Protein, 35g Carbohydrate, 3g Fat, 7g Fiber*

In your favorite bowl or 'to go' container, swirl the following.

1 cup non fat plain yogurt
1 squirt dijon mustard
½  scoop vanilla whey protein powder

Stir in the following.

3 oz or 1/2 large carrot
1 tablespoon raisins

TIP
Even better when its been chilled for a while!

**break sweat. don't break stride.**

# ☀ CINNAMON RAISIN BRAN MUFFINS
## (SUPER QUICK)

*Servings: 1*
*Per serving: 230cal, 23g Protein, 24.5g Carbohydrate, 3.4g Fiber, 4g Fat*
*Thanks to: Cathy Griffith*

Mix the following into small glass cereal bowl.

    1 scoop vanilla whey protein powder
    2 tablespoons oat flour (or oatbran)
    1 tablespoon all bran cereal
    1 tablespoon raisins
    1 tablespoon crushed walnuts
    ¼ teaspoon aluminum free baking soda
    ¼ teaspoon cinnamon
    pinch of preferred sweetener to taste
    ½ cup water

Microwave for 2 minutes.
Very moist and filling.

NOTE
Bran and nuts tend to settle to the bottom.

**plan meals. graze often.**

# COUNT CHOCOHOLIC CEREAL

*Servings: 1*

**WITH WHEY PROTEIN & COW'S MILK:**
*Per serving: 222cal, 20g Protein, 31g Carbohydrate, 3g Fat, 7g Fiber*

**WITH RICE PROTEIN & SOY MILK:**
*Per serving: 212cal, 16g Protein, 32g Carbohydrate, 3.5g Fat, 10g Fiber*

**WITH SOY PROTEIN & SOY MILK:**
*Per serving: 212cal, 21g Protein, 29g Carbohydrate, 2.5g Fat, 8g Fiber*

With child like thoughts, blend the following.

½ cup non fat milk or soy milk
½ scoop protein powder (chocolate or vanilla)
1-2 teaspoons unsweetened cocoa powder
pinch of preferred sweetener

Pour it over top of:

1 & ½ cups toasted oat cereal

NOTE
If you use **soy protein**, you may have to use more milk

INSPIRATION
Remember Count Chocula & Booberry Cereals? Follow
this same recipe with berry flavored Whey Protein for the
fitness version of "Booberry"

**break sweat. don't break stride.**

# ☀ CREAMSICLE SMOOTHIE

*Servings: 1*
*Per serving: 369 cal, 29g Protein, 60g Carbohydrate, 2.5g Fat, 4g Fiber*
*Thanks to: Michele Theoret*

Raise up onto your toes and mix the following with a blender.

    1 scoop vanilla whey
    1 banana
    ¾ cup orange juice
    1/2 cup fat free vanilla yogurt
    ice

# ☀ DAD'S COOKIE SMOOTHIE

*Servings: 1*
*Per serving: 320cal, 4g Fat, 35g Protein, 35g Carbohydrate, 5.3g Fiber*
*Thanks to: Michele Theoret*


Raise up onto your toes and mix the following with a blender.

  1 scoop vanilla whey
  1/3-cup oatmeal
  ½ banana
  1-cup skim milk or soy milk
  1/8 cup unsweetened coconut
  ½ capful coconut extract
  preferred sweetener to taste
  ice

# ☀ FROZEN YOGURT

Servings: 1

***WITH WHEY PROTEIN & COW'S YOGURT:***
*Per serving: 314 cal,, 34g Protein, 39g Carbohydrate, 3.3g Fat, 5gFiber*

***WITH RICE PROTEIN & SOY YOGURT/MILK:***
*Per serving: 303 cal, 28g Protein, 31g Carbohydrate, 8.8g Fat, 7gFiber*

***WITH HEMP PROTEIN & SOY YOGURT/MILK:***
*Per serving: 323 cal, 27g Protein, 32g Carbohydrate, 11g Fat, 7gFiber*

Raise up onto your toes and mix the following with a blender.

   1 scoop protein powder (any flavor)
   ½ frozen banana
   1/4 cup non fat milk or soy milk
   6 non fat plain yogurt ice cubes

NOTE
Feel free to play with the flavors of your frozen yogurt!

# ☾☀ HEMP MEETS HUMMUS

*Servings: 1*
*Per serving: 350 cal, 21g Protein, 49g Carbohydrate, 11g Fat, 15g Fiber*

Smoosh the following in your blender or food processor.

    1 cup cooked garbanzo beans, drained
    1 tablespoon hemp, grapeseed or olive oil

Keep blending and add the following.

    ½ scoop hemp protein powder
    couple squirts of lemon juice
    2 cloves garlic, crushed
    your favorite spices (perhaps fresh cilantro!)

Chill in the fridge for a while.
Use it as a dip for the following.

    2 cups of your favorite raw veggies

**break sweat. don't break stride.**

# ☀🕐 HOMEMADE PROTEIN BARS
## (BAKED)
*Servings: 6*

*Per serving: 211cal, 19g Protein, 24g Carbohydrate, 4g Fat, 3g Fiber*
*Thanks to: Cathy Griffith*

Preheat oven to 325.
Balance on one foot and stir the following in a big bowl.

   4 scoops chocolate whey protein powder
   ½ cup rolled oats
   ½ cup raisins
   ½ cup nonfat non fat milk or soy milk or soy
   ½ cup applesauce
   1/3 cup egg beaters or 2-3 egg whites
   2 tablespoons almond butter
   ¼ -1/3 cup water


Spray a brownie pan with cooking spray.
Pour mixture into pan - spread evenly.

Bake approx 20 minutes.
Cool Slightly - Cut into 6 bars.
Once cooked wrap individually w/ Saran Wrap.
Store in the fridge.

**plan meals. graze often.**

#  HOMEMADE BARS (NO-BAKE)

*Servings: 6*
*Per serving: 86cal, 18g Protein, 18g Carbohydrate, 4.5g Fat, 2g Fiber*
*Thanks to: Cathy Griffith*

Mix the following with a fork.

- 4 scoops whey protein powder
- ½ cup rolled oats
- ¼ cup raisins
- 2 tablespoons almond butter
- 1/3 cup water

Spread into shallow pan.
Place in Fridge.
Cut into 6 equal squares.

# ☀ JELLO DELIGHT (as a meal!)

*Servings: 1*

**WITH WHEY PROTEIN & COW'S MILK:**
*Per serving: 318 cal, 33.5g Protein, 32g Carbohydrate, 6g Fat, 5g Fiber*

**WITH RICE PROTEIN & SOY MILK:**
*Per serving: 282 cal, 26g Protein, 32g Carbohydrate, 6.5g Fat, 11g Fiber*

**WITH HEMP PROTEIN & SOY MILK:**
*Per serving: 302 cal, 25g Protein, 33g Carbohydrate, 8.5g Fat, 11gFiber*

Raise up onto your toes and mix the following with a blender.

   1 scoop vanilla protein powder
   ½ frozen banana
   1 cup non fat milk or soy milk

Pour over top of:

   ½ package of light jello (prepared into jello)

Top with:

   1 tablespoon hemp hearts (seeds)

**plan meals. graze often.**

# ✳ JORDAN'S SPORTY DESSERT MEAL

Servings: 1

*WITH WHEY PROTEIN & COW'S YOGURT:*
*Per serving: 345cal, 31g Protein, 49g Carbohydrate, 2.5g Fat, 10g Fiber*

*WITH RICE PROTEIN & SOY YOGURT:*
*Per serving: 336cal, 26g Protein, 41g Carbohydrate, 8g Fat, 12g Fiber*

*WITH SOY PROTEIN & SOY YOGURT:*
*Per serving: 336cal, 36g Protein, 35g Carbohydrate, 6g Fat, 8g Fiber*

Balance on one foot and stir the following in a bowl.

- 1 cup yogurt or soy yogurt
- 1 scoop protein powder
- 1 tablespoon of "no sugar added" strawberry jam
- 1 cup of mixed fruit (diced) apple, bannana, pear

¼ cup shredded wheat cereal (crumbled)

NOTE
If you are not going to eat it right away, then keep the
Shredded Wheat out. It gets soggy if it sits for a while.

INSPIRATION
This was a high request snack for my 11 year old step-son
who loves to play sports!

**break sweat. don't break stride.**

# ☾☀ KERI'S MOVIE NIGHT POPCORN

Servings: 1

***WITH WHEY PROTEIN & COW'S MILK:***
*Per serving: 326cal, 35g Protein, 47g Carbohydrate, 2.5g Fat, 11g Fiber*

***WITH RICE PROTEIN & SOY MILK:***
*Per serving: 290cal, 27g Protein, 47g Carbohydrate, 4.5g Fat, 17g Fiber*

***WITH HEMP PROTEIN & SOY MILK:***
*Per serving: 310cal, 26g Protein, 48g Carbohydrate, 6.5g Fat, 16g Fiber*

Mix the following in a blender (it's your drink).

    1 scoop whey or rice or hemp protein powder (any flavor)
    1 cup non fat milk or soy milk

Prepare your popcorn:

    5 cups of air-popped popcorn
    spritz with oil
    shake on dill seasoning (low sodium)

Play with the spices on the popcorn…there are tones of options.

    - hot sauce and curry powder
    - bragg's amino acids and nutritional yeast
    - Italian  or greek seasoning with fresh lemonsqueeze
    - maple syurup and sea salt
    - pizza seasoning spices

NOTES
If you choose to use Hemp Protein for your drink, you
might want to add some sweetener.

**plan meals.  graze often.**

# ☀🚗 LAZY MAN'S TREAT

*Servings: 1*
*Thanks to Darren Greenfield*

**WITH WHEY PROTEIN & COW'S YOGURT:**
*Per serving: 315cal, 36g Protein, 36g Carbohydrate, 4.5g Fat, 7g Fiber*

**WITH RICE PROTEIN & SOY YOGURT:**
*Per serving: 295cal, 30g Protein, 39g Carbohydrate, 5.5g Fat, 12g Fiber*

**WITH HEMP PROTEIN & SOY YOGURT:**
*Per serving: 315cal, 29g Protein, 39g Carbohydrate, 7.5g Fat, 11g Fiber*

In your favorite bowl or 'to go' container, swirl the following.

    1 cup nonfat plain yogurt or soy yogurt
    1 scoop protein powder (any flavor)
    ¼ cup rolled oats or ½ cup shredded wheat cereal

NOTE
If you choose to use hemp protein for a nice nutty flavor,
you might also want to add preferred sweetener.

TIP
If this is a snack you eat on a regular basis, then try pre-
roasting a quantity of oats in the oven with a spritz of your
favorite oil!

**break sweat. don't break stride.**

# 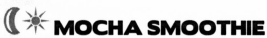 MOCHA SMOOTHIE

*Servings: 1*

**WITH WHEY PROTEIN & COW'S MILK:**
*Per serving: 206 cal, 29g Protein, 17g Carbohydrate, 1g Fat, 1g Fiber*

**WITH RICE PROTEIN & SOY MILK:**
*Per serving: 170 cal, 21g Protein, 17g Carbohydrate, 2g Fat, 7g Fiber*

**WITH HEMP PROTEIN & SOY MILK:** *(tastes best with Mate)*
*Per serving: 190 cal, 20g Protein, 18g Carbohydrate, 4g Fat, 7g Fiber*

Raise up onto your toes and mix the following with a blender.

   1 scoop chocolate protein powder
   6 coffee or yerba mate (dark roast) or Krakus ice cubes
   1 cup non fat milk or soy milk

NOTE
Instead of coffee icecubes you may also use regular ice-cubes with powdered coffee.

NOTE
If you would like a break from coffee try Krakus. It is a caffeine-free coffee flavored powder - great for mocha smoothies at midnight!

TIP
If you like this recipe, it would be a good idea to keep a tray of coffee or Yerba Mate dark roast or Krakus ice cubes in the freezer.

**plan meals.  graze often.**

# ☀ PEANUT BUTTER WRAP

*Servings: 1*
*Thanks to Lee Mein*

**WITH WHEY PROTEIN:**
*Per serving: 381cal, 22g Protein, 48g Carbohydrate, 10g Fat, 4g Fiber*

**WITH RICE PROTEIN:**
*Per serving: 371cal, 19g Protein, 49g Carbohydrate, 11g Fat, 6.5g Fiber*

Smoosh the following in a bowl with a wooden spoon.

    1 ½ tablespoons Natural Peanut Butter
    ½ scoop Whey Protein Powder (vanilla)
    1 teaspoon Ground Flax Meal

Spread on to:

    1 whole wheat tortilla
    Iceberg lettuce leaves

Roll and eat.

NOTE
The iceberg lettuce gives just enough moisture for the peanut butter/whey combo so it doesn't stick to the roof of your mouth!

# ✳ PROTEIN PANCAKES

*Servings: 1*
*Per serving: 382 cal, 40g Protein, 32.5g Carbohydrate, 5.1g Fat, 7g Fiber*
*Thanks to Kristen Reisinger*

Raise up onto your toes and mix the following with a blender.

½ scoop whey protein powder (strawberry is best)
2-3 egg whites
1/4 cup 1% cottage cheese
3 ounces extra firm low fat tofu
1/2 cup old fashioned oatmeal

Pour into non-stick med-high heat pan.
Cook like pancakes flipping when bubbles appear.

# ☀ PROTEIN SPIKED OATMEAL SERIES

TIP
When you cook the oatmeal (microwave or stove top) make it a little more runny than usual (use more water).

When you stir in the whey protein it will soak up most of the extra moisture. You will also want to make sure it is cooled down a bit PRIOR to adding the whey powder. When whey is heated, it has the tendency to get yucky!

NOTE
The combinations of rice/hemp protein and soy milk is for creating a Vegan meal. I didn't include Soy Protein as an option because it tends to make the oatmeal super thick and the flavor is not the best.

## A: Basic Oatmeal
*Servings: 1*

**WITH WHEY PROTEIN & COW'S MILK:**
*Per serving: 335cal, 35g Protein, 39g Carbohydrate, 5g Fat, 10g Fiber*

**WITH RICE PROTEIN & SOY MILK:**
*Per serving: 315cal, 28g Protein, 41g Carbohydrate, 6g Fat, 15g Fiber*

MAKE YOUR OATMEAL

Bring to a boil ½ cup water (+/-).
Stir in ½ cup (dry measure) rolled oats.
Cover and let thicken for approx. 5 minutes.

Balance on one foot and stir in the following.

2 teaspoons ground flax meal
1 scoop whey protein or rice protein (your favorite flavor)
½ cup non fat milk or soy milk

**break sweat. don't break stride.**

# B: Apple Cider Oatmeal

*Servings: 1*

**WITH WHEY PROTEIN :**
*Per serving: 290cal, 31g Protein, 33g Carbohydrate, 5g Fat, 9g Fiber*

**WITH RICE PROTEIN :**
*Per serving: 270cal, 25g Protein, 35g Carbohydrate, 6g Fat, 14g Fiber*

MAKE YOUR OATMEAL
   Bring to a boil ½ cup water (+/-)
   Stir in ½ cup (dry measure) rolled oats
   1 drop vanilla extract
   1 pinch cinnamon
   Cover and let thicken for approx. 5 minutes

Balance on one foot and stir in the following.

   1 scoop whey or rice protein (vanilla)
   1 splash of apple cider vinegar
   2 teaspoons ground flax meal

# C: Banana Bread Oatmeal

*Servings: 1*

**WITH WHEY PROTEIN & COW'S MILK:**
*Per serving: 365cal, 37g Protein, 39g Carbohydrate, 7.5g Fat, 12g Fiber*

**WITH RICE PROTEIN & SOY MILK:**
*Per serving: 345cal, 30g Protein, 41g Carbohydrate, 8.5g Fat, 17g Fiber*

MAKE YOUR OATMEAL

Bring to a boil ½ cup water (+/-).
Stir in ½ cup (dry measure) rolled oats.
Cover and let thicken for approx. 5 minutes.

Balance on one foot and stir in the following.

2 teaspoons ground flax meal
2 teaspoons hemp hearts (seeds)
1-2 drops of banana extract
1 dash allspice
1 dash nutmeg
1 dash cinnamon
1 scoop whey or rice protein (vanilla)
½ cup non fat milk or soy milk

**break sweat. don't break stride.**

# D: Scott's Nutty Oats

*Servings: 1*
*Thanks to Scott McKenzie*

**WITH WHEY PROTEIN & COW'S MILK:**
*Per serving: 417cal, 40g Protein, 42g Carbohydrate, 12g Fat, 13g Fiber*

**WITH RICE PROTEIN & SOY MILK:**
*Per serving: 407cal, 34g Protein, 44g Carbohydrate, 13g Fat, 17g Fiber*

MAKE YOUR OATMEAL

Bring to a boil ½ cup water (+/-).
Stir in ½ cup (dry measure) rolled oats.
Cover and let thicken for approx. 5 minutes.

Balance on one foot and stir in the following.

1 dash cinnamon
1 tablespoon unsweetened coconut
½ ounce (5-7 nuts) of unsalted mixed nuts
1 scoop protein powder (vanilla)
½ cup non fat milk or soy milk

**plan meals. graze often.**

# E: Chet's Ice Cream Oats

*Servings: 1*
*Thanks to Chet Neyhart*

**WITH WHEY PROTEIN & COW'S MILK:**
*Per serving: 335cal, 35g Protein, 39g Carbohydrate, 5g Fat, 10g Fiber*

**WITH RICE PROTEIN & SOY MILK:**
*Per serving: 315cal, 28g Protein, 41g Carbohydrate, 6g Fat, 15g Fiber*

MAKE YOUR OATMEAL

Bring to a boil ½ cup water (+/-).
Stir in ½ cup (dry measure) rolled oats.
Cover and let thicken for approx. 5 minutes.

Raise up onto your toes and mix the following with a blender.

1 scoop whey protein (vanilla)
approx 8 ice cubes
½ cup non fat milk or soy milk

Pour the mock icecream mixture over your oats.

# F: Warm Apple Pie & Ice Cream
*Servings: 1*

**WITH WHEY PROTEIN & COW'S MILK:**
*Per serving: 352cal, 31g Protein, 50g Carbohydrate, 4g Fat, 10g Fiber*

**WITH RICE PROTEIN & SOY MILK:**
*Per serving: 332cal, 25g Protein, 52g Carbohydrate, 5g Fat, 15g Fiber*

MAKE YOUR OATMEAL

Bring to a boil ½ cup water (+/-).
Stir in ½ cup (dry measure) rolled oats.
Cover and let thicken for approx. 5 minutes.

Raise up onto your toes and mix the following with a blender.

2 teaspoons ground flax meal
1 pinch cinnamon
½ apple (diced or sliced)
1 scoop whey protein (vanilla)
½ frozen banana
½ cup non fat milk or soy milk

Pour the mock icecream mixture over your oats.

**plan meals. graze often.**

# G: Cinnamon Bun Oatmeal

*Servings: 1*

**WITH WHEY PROTEIN & COW'S MILK:**
*Per serving: 375cal, 34g Protein, 38g Carbohydrate, 10.6g Fat, 9g Fiber*

**WITH RICE PROTEIN & SOY MILK:**
*Per serving: 355cal, 28g Protein, 40g Carbohydrate, 11.5g Fat, 14g Fiber*

MAKE YOUR OATMEAL

Bring to a boil ½ cup water (+/-).
Stir in ½ cup (dry measure) rolled oats.
Cover and let thicken for approx. 5 minutes.

Balance on one foot and stir in the following.

1 teaspoon vanilla extract
2 pinches of cinnamon
1 molly mcbutter or butter buds
1 scoop whey protein (vanilla)
½ cup non fat milk or soy milk
2 teaspoons hemp, udo's, or grapeseed oil

# Double Chocolate Oatmeal
*Servings: 1*

**WITH WHEY PROTEIN & COW'S MILK:**
*Per serving: 347cal, 36g Protein, 42g Carbohydrate, 6g Fat, 12g Fiber*

**WITH RICE PROTEIN & SOY MILK:**
*Per serving: 327cal, 30g Protein, 44g Carbohydrate, 7g Fat, 17g Fiber*

**WITH 1T PEANUT BUTTER & WHEY PROTEIN & COW'S MILK:**
*Per serving: 448 cal, 40g Protein, 46g Carbohydrate, 14g Fat, 13g Fiber*

**WITH 1T PEANUT BUTTER & RICE PROTEIN & SOY MILK:**
*Per serving: 428 cal, 34g Protein, 48g Carbohydrate, 15g Fat, 18g Fiber*


MAKE YOUR OATMEAL

Bring to a boil ½ cup water (+/-).
Stir in ½ cup (dry measure) rolled oats.
Cover and let thicken for approx. 5 minutes.

Balance on one foot and stir in the following.

1-2 teaspoons unsweetened cocoa
pinch of preferred sweetener
2 teaspoons ground flax meal
1 scoop whey protein (chocolate)
½ cup non fat milk or soy milk

# Maple Walnut Oats
*Servings: 1*

***WITH WHEY PROTEIN & COW'S MILK:***
*Per serving: 383cal, 37g Protein, 40g Carbohydrate, 10g Fat, 11g Fiber*

***WITH RICE PROTEIN & SOY MILK:***
*Per serving: 363cal, 31g Protein, 42g Carbohydrate, 11g Fat, 16g Fiber*

MAKE YOUR OATMEAL

Bring to a boil ½ cup water (+/-).
Stir in ½ cup (dry measure) rolled oats.
Cover and let thicken for approx. 5 minutes.

Balance on one foot and stir in the following.

couple drops of maple extract
1 scoop whey protein (vanilla)
1 tablespoon (ground or crushed walnuts)
½ cup non fat milk or soy milk

# H: Fresh Berries & Oatmeal

*Servings: 1*

**WITH WHEY PROTEIN & COW'S MILK:**
*Per serving: 377cal, 35g Protein, 50g Carbohydrate, 5g Fat, 11.5g Fiber*

**WITH RICE PROTEIN & SOY MILK:**
*Per serving: 357cal, 29g Protein, 52g Carbohydrate, 6g Fat, 16.5g Fiber*

MAKE YOUR OATMEAL

Bring to a boil ½ cup water (+/-).
Stir in ½ cup (dry measure) rolled oats.
Cover and let thicken for approx. 5 minutes.

Balance on one foot and stir in the following.

2 teaspoons ground flax meal
1 scoop whey protein (chocolate or vanilla or berry blend)
½ cup berries
½ cup non fat milk or soy milk

# ☀ RICE PUDDING

Servings: 1

***WITH WHEY PROTEIN & COW'S MILK:***
*Per serving: 274cal, 28g Protein, 34g Carbohydrate, 2g Fat, 4g Fiber*

***WITH RICE PROTEIN & SOY MILK:***
*Per serving: 254cal, 22g Protein, 36g Carbohydrate, 3g Fat, 9g Fiber*

***WITH SOY PROTEIN & SOY MILK:***
*Per serving: 254cal, 32g Protein, 30g Carbohydrate, 1g Fat, 5g Fiber*

With care, combine the following in a low-heat pot.

½ cup cooked Rice
½ cup non fat milk or soy milk
1 pinch Cinnamon
Couple drops of pure vanilla extract

Stir and do not bring to a boil.
Once it is warm (not hot), stir in the following.

1 scoop Protein Powder (vanilla)

NOTE
Great quick recipe when you have some pre-cooked rice.
Eat it warm or cold.

TIPS
Multiply the servings and make a big pot all at once.

It's even better when it has sat in the fridge over night.

Try it with some raisins too. Add some carb grams.

HINT
Try quinoa instead of rice.

**break sweat. don't break stride.**

# ✳ TRIO OF CHOCOLATE SMOOTHIES
## (FOR THOSE CANDY BAR CRAVINGS)

## A: Chocolate Caramel Smoothie
*Servings: 1*

**WITH WHEY PROTEIN & COW'S MILK:**
*Per serving: 293 cal, 31g Protein, 35g Carbohydrate, 3g Fat, 4g Fiber*

**WITH RICE PROTEIN & SOY MILK:**
*Per serving: 257 cal, 23g Protein, 34.5g Carbohydrate, 4g Fat, 10g Fiber*

Raise up onto your toes and mix the following with a blender.

- 1 scoop chocolate protein powder
- ½ frozen banana
- 1 cup non fat milk or soy milk
- 1 tablespoon caramel or butterscotch pudding powder

Stir in:

- 1 tablespoon unsweetened carob chips

# B: Chocolate Caramel Pecan Smoothie
*Servings: 1*

**WITH WHEY PROTEIN & COW'S MILK:**
*Per serving: 341 cal, 33g Protein, 36g Carbohydrate, 8g Fat, 5g Fiber*

**WITH RICE PROTEIN & SOY MILK:**
*Per serving: 305 cal, 25g Protein, 35.5g Carbohydrate, 9g Fat, 11g Fiber*

Raise up onto your toes and mix the following with a blender.

- 1 scoop chocolate protein powder
- ½ frozen banana
- 1 cup non fat milk or soy milk
- 1 tablespoon caramel or butterscotch pudding powder

Stir in:

- 1 tablespoon of crushed pecans.

# C: Chocolate Peanut Butter Smoothie
*Servings: 1*

**WITH WHEY PROTEIN & COW'S MILK:**
*Per serving: 394 cal, 35g Protein, 39g Carbohydrate, 11g Fat, 5g Fiber*

**WITH RICE PROTEIN & SOY MILK:**
*Per serving: 358 cal, 27g Protein, 38g Carbohydrate, 12g Fat, 11g Fiber*

Raise up onto your toes and mix the following with a blender.

- 1 scoop chocolate protein powder
- ½ frozen banana
- 1 cup non fat milk or soy milk
- 1 tablespoon caramel or butterscotch pudding powder

Stir in:

- 1 tablespoon of chunky peanut butter

**break sweat. don't break stride.**

# ☀🕐 TASTY ORGASMIC DELIGHTS
## (YUMMY NO-BAKE SQUARES)

*Servings: 4*
*Per serving: 285cal, 27g Protein, 27g Carbohydrate, 9g Fat, 9g Fiber*
*Thanks to Jay Solomon*

Playfully toss the following in a big bowl.

    2 scoops of soy protein powder
    ½ scoop hemp protein powder
    1 tablespoon ground flax meal
    3 tablespoons unsweetened cocoa or carob powder

With a strong wood spoon, stir while pouring in:

    2 cups soy milk

Keep stirring until you have a thick "cookie dough" consistency
and there are no more lumps of pure powder.
Flex your biceps and stir in the following.

    3 tablespoons natural peanut butter (jay likes skippy!)
    1 cup rolled oats

The batter will be really thick (you may have to play with the ingredients and maybe some water to get it right).

Scoop the mixture into a cassorole dish, level it with your spoon,
place it in the fridge for at least 4 hours.

Keep refrigerated until you want to eat it.
Divide into 4 equal portions.

> TIP
> Instead of spreading mixture into a cassorole dish, you
> can roll into little balls and place on a wax paper sheet and
> place them in the freezer.

**plan meals. graze often.**

# ☾ TEA LATTE SMOOTHIE
*Servings: 1*

***WITH WHEY PROTEIN & COW'S MILK:***
*Per serving: 206 cal, 29g Protein, 17g Carbohydrate, 1g Fat, 1g Fiber*

***WITH RICE PROTEIN & SOY MILK:***
*Per serving: 170 cal, 21g Protein, 17g Carbohydrate, 2g Fat, 7g Fiber*

***WITH HEMP PROTEIN & SOY MILK:***
*Per serving: 190 cal, 20g Protein, 18g Carbohydrate, 4g Fat, 7g Fiber*

Raise up onto your toes and mix the following with a blender.

  1 scoop vanilla protein powder
  6 ice cubes
  ½ cup non fat milk or soy milk
  ½ of strong brewed and cooled tea (black, green, herbal, etc)

> TIP
> Some of my favorite teas for this meal: Indian Chai, Rooi-
> bos, Jasmine Green, Morracan Mint, or Lavender. Fruit
> teas also work really well.

**break sweat. don't break stride.**

# 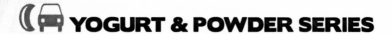 YOGURT & POWDER SERIES

## A: Simple Whey Time
*Servings: 1*
*Per serving: 240 cal, 31g Protein, 23g Carbohydrate, 3g Fat, 4g Fiber*

In your favorite bowl or 'to go' container, swirl the following.

   1 cup plain nonfat yogurt
   1 scoop whey protein powder (pick your flavor)

Done!

## Cake Batter (vegan)
*Servings: 1*

***WITH COW'S YOGURT:***
*Per serving: 230cal, 25g Protein, 28g Carbohydrate, 4g Fat, 9g Fiber*

***WITH SOY YOGURT:***
*Per serving: 244cal, 26g Protein, 17g Carbohydrate, 8.5g Fat, 6g Fiber*

In your favorite bowl or 'to go' container, swirl the following.

   1 cup plain nonfat yogurt or soy yogurt
   1 scoop rice protein powder (vanilla or chocolate)
   sprinkle or ½ tsp. of pudding mix powder (vanilla or chocolate)

> NOTE
> The rice protein powder turns out more like cake batter.
> Feel free to play with the flavors of pudding. It can also
> work without the pudding.

**plan meals. graze often.**

# B: Green Power (vegan)
*Servings: 1*

**WITH COW'S YOGURT:**
*Per serving: 270cal, 26g Protein, 26.5g Carbohydrate, 8g Fat, 10g Fiber*

**WITH SOY YOGURT:**
*Per serving: 284cal, 27g Protein, 16.5g Carbohydrate, 12g Fat, 7g Fiber*

In your favorite bowl or 'to go' container, swirl the following.

  1 cup plain nonfat yogurt or soy yogurt
  1 scoop hemp protein powder
  2 teaspoons hemp hearts (seeds)
  you may want to add preferred sweetener to this one

Get your essential fatty acids and good bacterias all in one snack!

# C: Cookie Dough (vegan)
*Servings: 1*

**WITH COW'S YOGURT:**
*Per serving: 255cal, 36g Protein, 23g Carbohydrate, 3.5g Fat, 7g Fiber*

**WITH SOY YOGURT:**
*Per serving: 269cal, 37g Protein, 13g Carbohydrate, 8g Fat, 4g Fiber*

In your favorite bowl or 'to go' container, swirl the following.

  1 cup plain nonfat yogurt or soy yogurt
  1 scoop plain soy protein powder
  couple drops of vanilla extract
  pinch of preferred sweetener
  1 tablespoon carob chips

**break sweat. don't break stride.**

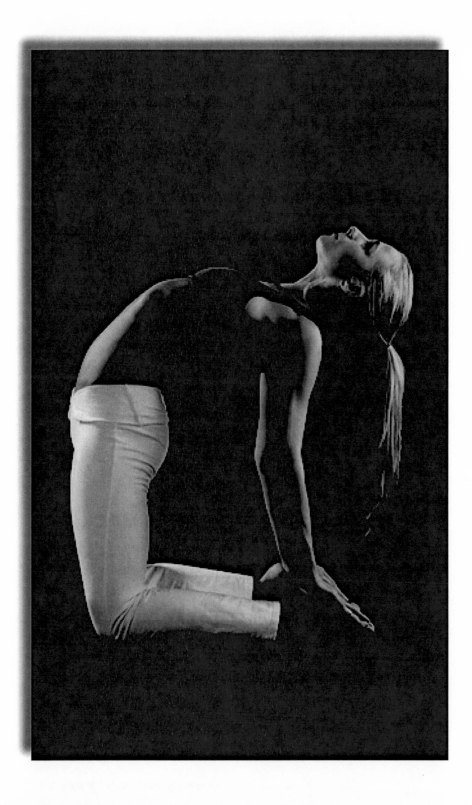

# BodyArtist

## Kristi Lees

Yoga Teacher and Fitness Enthusiast

Sometimes I just feel so bound up in the physical body, so restricted. Physical activity whether it be dance, circus training, cardio, yoga, strength training etc gives me a way to break free from that; to get out of my body, to feel its lightness ... even if sometimes it is just momentarily.

It's taken awhile to get there because training used to be a means that binded me. When I was going through an eating disorder and the years that followed, training was about controlling the body - not liberating myself through it.

# What to do with:
# NO ANIMAL PRODUCTS

## Tempeh
### (fermented soybeans)

## Veggie Burgers
### (calculated from Boca brand)

# ☾ BASIC VEGGIE BURGER STIR-FRY

*Servings: 1*
*per serving: 197 cal, 20g Protein, 28g Carbohydrate, 1.5g Fat, 12g Fiber*

With care, toss the following in a medium-heat deep dish pan.

  1 veggie burger (cut into chunks)
  10 oz or couple handfuls of oriental veggie mix
  1-2 sliced cloves of fresh garlic (or teaspoon of pre-minced)
  1 slice fresh ginger root (minced)
  splash of bragg's amino acids
  splash of water
  1 pinch preferred sweetener
  your favorite spices

Stir occasionally for a couple of minutes…until the veggies are warm but still crisp. Finish with a squeeze of fresh lemon or lime.

NOTE
This is the basic recipe….from here just play with  different veggies and spices. You could have different dishes every-day just from this one recipe.

# ☾ BASIC TOMATO TEMPEH SKILLET
*Servings: 1*

**JUST THE SAUCE:**
*per serving: 192cal, 17g Protein, 23g Carbohydrate, 5.2g Fat, 10g Fiber*

**POURED OVER 1/2 medium SPAGEHETTI SQUASH:**
*per serving: 276cal, 19g Protein, 43g Carbohydrate, 6g Fat, 14g Fiber*

With care, toss the following in a medium-heat deep dish pan.

½ cup tempeh
2 tablespoons tomato paste
½ cup water
squirt of bragg's amino acids
handful of mushrooms (sliced)
handful of broccoli (chopped)
green onion or scallion (chopped)
1-2 cloves of garlic
splash of rice vinegar
squirt of hot sauce
pinch of oregano
pinch of basil

Balance on one foot and stir.
Cover and allow the flavors to dance for a little bit.

TIP
Play with different veggie and spice combinations.

**break sweat. don't break stride.**

# ☾ ☀ 🚗 BRANDIE'S SIMPLE VEG CHILI

*Servings: 1*
*per serving: 221 cal, 24g Protein, 38.5g Carbohydrate, 2.5g Fat, 6g Fiber*
*Thanks to Brandie Vander Hiede*

With care, toss the following in a medium-heat deep dish pan.
Or stir it all into a 'to go' container to heat on the road.

    1/3 cup ground veggie
    1 cup cooked mixed vegetables
        (corn, peas, carrots, green beans)
    1/2 cup chunky tomato sauce
    1-2 shakes mexcian spices

# ☾ VEGGIE BURGER & GREENS

*Servings: 1*
*per serving: 256 cal, 27g Protein, 37g Carbohydrate 2g Fat, 14g Fiber*

### ADD 1/4 OF LARGE OR 1/2 SMALL AVOCADO:
*348 cal, 28g Protein, 41g Carbohydrate 10.5g Fat, 18g Fiber*

With care, toss the following in a medium-heat deep dish pan.

    1 veggie burger (diced)
    ¼ onion (chopped)
    handful of mushrooms (diced)
    1 small zucchini
    handful or approx 8 oz broccoli (chopped)
    1 pinches fresh parsley
    1 pinch curry
    1 tablespoon nutritional yeast (optional)

Playfully toss the following in a big bowl.

    2-3 handfuls of mixed salad greens
    1 fresh roma tomato or a couple cherry tomatoes
    ¼ of large avocado (optional)

Pour the warm pan mixture onto the salad.

**break sweat. don't break stride.**

# ❰ CARROTS & VEGGIE BURGER

*Servings: 1*
*per serving: 219cal, 19g Protein, 26g Carbohydrate, 5.6g Fat, 11g Fiber*

Boil the following for about 5-7 minutes.

   1 medium sized (6oz) Carrot (sliced)

Then drain the water out of the pot and add

   1 Veggie Burger (chopped)

Balance on one foot and stir for a minute, then add:

   1 teaspoon hemp, flax, udo's, or mct Oil
   1 tablespoon Nutritional Yeast

> TIP
> This is a good recipe to double/triple as it will store well in the fridge for a couple of days.

**plan meals.  graze often.**

# ❲ CURRY CABBAGE STIR-FRY

*Servings: 1*
*per serving: 255 cal, 21g Protein, 24g Carbohydrate 11g Fat, 12g Fiber*

With care, toss the following in a medium-heat deep dish pan.

    1 veggie burger
    1 handful of mushrooms (sliced) or about 3 med. mushrooms
    ¼ green bell pepper (sliced)
    1-2 cloves garlic (diced)
    1 small dash fennel
    1 pinch of curry
    1 pinch of corriander
    1 tablespoon raw pumpkin seeds

Balance on one foot and stir until the flavors dance.
Add the following and keep stiring for a minute until blended.

    2 cups shredded cabbage
    1 teaspoon coconut, hemp, grapeseed, or olive oil

**break sweat. don't break stride.**

# 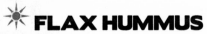 FLAX HUMMUS

*Servings: 2*
*per serving: 290 cal, 14g Protein, 45g Carbohydrate, 8.5g Fat, 12g Fiber*
*Thanks to Kristin Reisinger*

Raise up onto toes - blend the following with a food processor.

   1 cup cooked garbanzo beans (drained)

Once smooth, slowly add the following.

   2 tablespoons flax oil
   1/3 cup lemon juice
   2 cloves garlic (crushed)
   1 pinch cayenne pepper (or to taste)
   1 tablespoon chopped parsley

Let chill and use as a dip for:

   2 cups of your favorite raw veggies

# ☀ GOTTA HAVE BEANS & RICE

*Servings: 1*
*per serving: 198 cal, 8.5g Protein, 35g Carbohydrate, 4g Fat, 6g Fiber*

With care, toss the following in a medium-heat deep dish pan and stir.

2 tablespoons chopped onion
1 clove of garlic (chopped)

After a couple minutes, add the following and keep stirring.

   1/3 cup cooked rice
   ½ cup kidney beans
   ¼ cup lite, unsweetened coconut milk
   1 pinch of chili powder

Let the flavors blend for a couple minutes.

INSPIRATION
You can't have a Vegan section without at least one "beans & rice" recipe! The combination of "beans & rice" is the stereotypical vegan complete protein meal.

**break sweat. don't break stride.**

# ✳ GREEN BEANS & APPLESAUCE

*Servings: 1*
*per serving: 206 cal, 22g Protein, 31g Carbohydrate, 3.5g Fat, 7g Fiber*

With care, toss the following in a medium-heat deep dish pan.

   3/4 cup meatless veggie ground
   1-2 handfuls or 5 oz of cut green beans

Stir for a couple minutes until warmed, then add:

   1/4 cup unsweetened applesauce
   2 dashes of cinnamon
   1 teaspoon oil

Simmer for a minute or two and allow the flavors to dance.

TIP
Option to toss all the ingredients into a to go container and
eat it cold.

**plan meals.  graze often.**

# ☾ HOT SPINACH TEMPEH SALAD

*Servings: 1*
*per serving: 201 cal, 22g Protein, 36g Carbohydrate, 6g Fat, 23g Fiber*

With care, toss the following in a medium-heat deep dish pan.

    1 chopped tempeh pattie (lemon flavor if you can find it)
    handful or about 4 whole mushrooms (sliced)
    2 garlic cloves (sliced)
    ¾ oz rice vinegar
    splash of water
    1 pinch of dill
    1 pinch of mustard powder
    1 dash cayenne pepper
    squirt or squeeze of fresh lemon

Stir and let simmer on low until the spices smell divine.
Stir in:

    1 teaspoon coconut oil

Pour the warm mixture over the following.

    2-3 handfuls or 4 cups of baby spinach
    1 handful or 1 cup of beet greens (optional)
    1 tablespoon nutritional yeast

NOTE
You can substitute the tempeh patty for a boca patty or boca ground.

TIP
Spinach is a great source of iron for the vegan warrior.

**break sweat. don't break stride.**

# 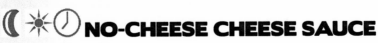 NO-CHEESE CHEESE SAUCE

Servings: 4
*Thanks to Kelly Phipps*

**JUST THE SAUCE**
*per serving:  176 cal, 11g Protein, 25g Carbohydrate, 6g Fat, 5g Fiber*

**WITH 2 CUPS OF STEAMED VEGGIES**
*(mushrooms, broccoli, cauliflower, carrots, etc.)*
*per serving: 226 cal, 13g Protein, 36g Carbohydrate, 6g Fat, 17g Fiber*

Steam the following for 15min. until it becomes soft.

1 medium butternut squash
(chopped in cubes - leave the skin on)

Raise up onto your toes and mix the following with a blender.

1/2 cup warm water
3 tbsp dijon mustard
3 tbsp tahini
3 tbsp tamari
1/2 cup nutritional yeast

Add steamed sqaush and continue to blend. You may want to either add a little more water or nutritional yeast flakes to desired creaminess/thickness.

Pour over lightly steamed veggies and add some pepper.

NOTE
This is recipe, unlike most in this book has a few ingredients you may have never heard of.

You will most likely need to go to the local "green grocery" to get these ingredients:

Tahini - sesame seed nut butter.

Tamari -  a vegan soy sauce.

**plan meals.  graze often.**

# ☀ PEPPER SWEET POTATO FRY

*Servings: 1*
*per serving: 204 cal, 16 g Protein, 30g Carbohydrate, 1.5g Fat, 8g Fiber*

With care, toss the following in a medium-heat deep dish pan.

   1-2 garlic cloves (sliced)
   ¼ onion (sliced or chopped)
   splash of water

Balance on one foot and stir for a minute or two, then add:

   1 veggie burger (chopped)
   1 cup sweet potato or yam (boiled in cubes)
   ¼ red bell pepper (sliced or chopped)
   ¼ to ½ green bell pepper (sliced or chopped)

Balance on the other foot and stir some more until everything is warm. Top with:

   squirt of bragg's liquid amino acids
   optional squeeze of fresh lime

**break sweat. don't break stride.**

# QUICK NUT SNACK SERIES

### 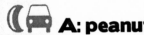 A: peanutbutter and carrots

*Servings: 1*
*per serving: 274 cal, 10g Protein, 26g Carbohydrate, 16.5g Fat, 8g Fiber*

1/2 small bag (6 oz) mini carrots
2 tablespoons natural peanut butter

###  B: fruit and nuts

*Servings: 1*
*per serving: 240 cal, 7.5g Protein, 26g Carbohydrat, 14.5g Fat, 7g Fiber*

1 whole fruit (banana, apple, orange, pear, peach, etc.)
1/2 small handful (1 oz) of unsalted mixed nuts and/or seeds

###  C: ants on a log

*Servings: 1*
*per serving: 244 cal, 5g Protein, 16g Carbohydrate, 18g Fat, 4g Fiber*

4 stalks of celery
2 tablespoons of almond butter
1 tablespoon raisins

###  D: peanutbutter and rice cakes

*Servings: 1*
*per serving: 272 cal, 10g Protein, 22g Carbohydrate, 16g Fat, 2g Fiber*

2 plain unsalted brown rice cakes
2 tablespoons of natural peanut butter

**plan meals. graze often.**

# ( ROMAINE TACOS

*Servings: 1*
*per serving: 296 cal, 35g Protein, 31g Carbohydrate, 11g Fat, 12g Fiber*


With care, toss the following in a medium-heat deep dish pan.

    1 cup ground veggie burger
    ¼ onion (chopped)
    1-2 handful of mushrooms (diced)
    1/2 green pepper (sliced)
    2 tablespoons salsa (or to taste)
    pinch of taco spice

Wash and separate:

    2-3 large romaine leafs (boats)

Scoop the warm mixture into the romaine boats and top with:

    ¼ large avocado (sliced)
    1 tablespoon nutritional yeast

# ☀🕐 SANDY'S SUPERB SOUP

*Servings: 3*
*per serving: 280 cal, 21g Protein, 38.5g Carbohydrate, 7g Fat, 14g Fat*

*Original invention by Sandy Cahoon*

Playfully toss the following into a big soup pot.

    2 cups tempeh
    1 medium onion (diced)
    2 cloves garlic (sliced)
    3 cups water
    3 stalks celery (chopped)
    1 medium carrot (sliced)
    1 cup mushrooms (sliced)
    1 large can diced tomatoes (drained & rinsed)
    couple squirts of bragg's amino acid's
    2 cups frozen green & yellow beans
    1 cup kidney beans (drained & rinsed)
    1 tablespoon chili powder (or to taste)
    1 teaspoon crushed chili peppers
    1 teaspoon basil

Simmer for a couple hours.  Stir every once in a while.

NOTE
Sandy is a mother of three who needs to make meals that the whole family will look forward to!

TIP
Great recipe to double or triple and put extra servings in the freezer.

**plan meals.  graze often.**

# ☾ SHEPARD'S PIE - Quick VEGAN STYLE

*Servings: 1*
*per serving: 205 cal, 32g Protein, 28g Carbohydrate 1g Fat, 9g Fiber*

With care, toss the following in a medium-heat deep dish pan.

> 1 cup meatless veggie burger ground
> 1 cup turnip (mashed)
> ¼ cup mixed veggies (peas, corn, carrot)
> ½ green onion (snipped) or dry chives
> 1 dash cayenne pepper
> 1 dash paprika
> 1 dash garlic powder (or real garlic cloves)

Balance on one foot and stir until warm. Top with:

> 1 tablespoon nutritional yeast

# ✳ SWEET POTATO Veggie burger TO GO

Servings: 1

*per serving:* 230 cal, 31g Protein, 34g Carbohydrate, 0.8g Fat, 8g Fiber

With care, toss the following in a medium-heat deep dish pan.
Or stir it all into a 'to go' container to heat on the road.

    1 cup meatless ground veggie burger
    ½ cup cooked sweet potato or yam (baked or boiled mashed)
    1 pinch cinnamon
    1 tablespoon nutritional yeast
    1 pinch preferred sweetener

# ☀ SLOPPY JOES

*Servings: 2*
**WITH THE BUN:**
*per serving: 201 cal, 21.5g Protein, 35g Carbohydrate, 0.8g Fat, 9g Fiber*

**WITHOUT THE BUN**
*per serving: 142 cal, 19g Protein, 24g Carbohydrate, 0.5g Fat, 6g Fiber*

With care, toss the following in a medium-heat deep dish pan.

¼ cup onion (diced)
1 medium zucchini, finely diced
1-2 cloves garlic, minced
splash of water

Stir for a minute or two, then add the following.

2 tablespoons tomato paste
1 cup water
1 cup ground meatless veggie burger
1/2 cup kidney beans (rinsed and drained)
1 pinch paprika
1 pinch basil
1 pinch chili powder
couple drops of liquid smoke (optional)
1 splash worsheire sauce
1 splash of tabasco (or to taste)
1 squirt ketchup
pinch of preferred sweetener
1 splash of cider vinegar

Simmer for about 5 minutes to let the flavors dance.
Scoop onto:

1 sprouted/grainy bun (optional)

NOTE
Great recipe to multiply - feed the family or make several
single meals for for the freezer.

**break sweat. don't break stride.**

# 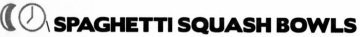 SPAGHETTI SQUASH BOWLS

*Servings: 2*
*per serving: 252 cal, 32g Protein, 40g Carbohydrate, 1.2g Fat, 10g Fiber*

With care, toss the following in a medium-heat deep dish pan.

½ red bell pepper
¼ cup onion
1-2 handful (1 cup) mushrooms (chopped)
1-2 handful (1 cup) broccoli (chopped)
2 cups vegan meatless ground veggie burger
1-2 pinch oregano
1-2 pinch thyme
1-2 pinch italian seasoning
1-2 squirts of bragg's liquid amino's

Stir for a couple minutes and let the flavors blend (5-10 minutes).
Scoop the mixture into:

1 medium spaghetti squash
(see front of book for instructions)

OPTION: top with Nutritional Yeast.

NOTE
The stir-fry filling can be used without the squash bowl, by
itself, or with rice.

# ☽ SIMPLE & SWEET STIR-FRY
*Servings: 1*
*per serving: 218 cal, 21g Protein, 27g Carbohydrate, 4.5g Fat, 12g Fiber*

With care, toss the following in a medium-heat deep dish pan.

- 1 veggie burger (chopped)
- 1-2 cloves garlic (sliced)
- 3-4 button mushrooms (sliced)
- 1 tablespoon sliced almonds
- 1 cup brocolli (chopped)
- ¾ cup water
- 2 cups shredded cabbage mix
- 1-2 splash of rice vinegar
- 1 pinch preferred sweetener

Stir and simmer until the flavors invite your taste buds and the cabbage is still a little bit firm.

**break sweat. don't break stride.**

# ( TOMATO & ZUCCHINI SKILLET

*Servings: 1*
*per serving: 331 cal, 26g Protein, 37g Carbohydrate, 10g Fat, 16g Fiber*

With care, toss the following in a high-heat deep dish pan.

  1 cup tempeh (chopped)
  1 cup cherry tomatoes (halved)
  1 medium to large zucchini (chopped or shredded)
  2 tablespoons tomato paste
  ¾ cup water
  ½ small onion (diced)
  1-3 cloves garlic (sliced)
  1 teaspoon paprika

Bring to a boil.
In a jar, shake the following.
While you're there, shake your hips too!

  1 teaspoon cornstarch
  1/8 cup water

Stir and pour the cornstarch into the pan until it thickens.

# ☾ TEMPEH DIP OR SPREAD
*Servings: 3*

**JUST THE DIP:**
*per serving: 185cal, 14g Protein, 8.5g Carbohydrate, 7g Fat, 5g Fiber*

**WITH 2 cups of RAW VEGGIES:**
*per serving: 235cal, 16g Protein, 19.5g Carbohydrate, 7g Fat, 8g Fiber*

With care, toss the following in a medium-heat pan.

  2 cups of tempeh
  2-3 cloves garlic
  2 teaspoons oil

Raise up onto your toes and mix the following with a blender.

  ¼ cup water
  ¼ cup of balsamic vinegar
  squirt of bragg's amino acids
  pinch fresh parsley
  pinch fresh basil
  pinch of paprika
  pinch of tumeric
  pinch of cumin
  (feel free to play and substitute the spices to suit your tastes)

Stir the following into the blended mixture.

  ½ cup onions (diced)
  ¼ cup black olives (diced)

NOTE
If you are using it as a spread, refridgerate for at least
two hours. If you are using it as a dip you may use it right
away.

**break sweat. don't break stride.**

# ☀ VEGAN FRENCH TOAST

*Servings: 2*
*per serving: 237 cal, 19.5g Protein, 34.5g Carbohydrate, 2g Fat, 6g Fiber*
*Thanks to Kristin Reisinger*

Raise up onto your toes and mix the following with a blender until it resembles the consistancy of two beaten eggs.

    1/2 pkg. soft tofu
    1/4 cup of soy milk or rice milk
    1 teaspoon vanilla extract
    1 teaspoon cinnamon
    1/4 cup of water

Pour the liquid mixture onto a plate and dip the following in it.

    4 slices sprouted/grainy bread

Place in a medium-heat iron skillet until golden brown, flip once.

**plan meals. graze often.**

# ◖ VEGAN POPCORN SERIES

## A: bragg'n with yeast

*Servings: 2*

*per serving: 235 cal, 8g Protein, 33g Carbohydrate, 9g Fiber*
*Thanks to Kelly Phipps*

Prepare your popcorn:
   10 cups of air-popped popcorn

Spritz or pour on:
   1 tablespoon of oil
   1-3 squirts of bragg's amino acids

Shake on:
   2 tablespoons nutritional yeast

## B: peanut butter popcorn

*Servings: 2*

*per serving: 256 cal, 9g Protein, 35g Carbohydrate, 10g Fat, 7g Fiber*

Prepare your popcorn:
   10 cups of air-popped popcorn

Melt the following:
   2 tablespoons natural peanut butter

**break sweat. don't break stride.**

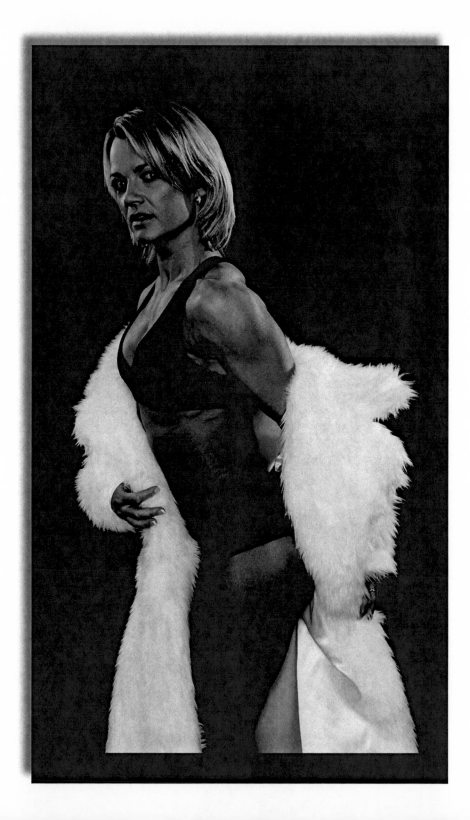

# BodyArtist

## Eva Sefcova

E.V.A. Fitness
WNSO Personal Trainer and Sports Nutritionist
Professional FAME Fitness Model

Photo by: David Ford

Fitness and a healthy lifestyle should be an essential part of everyone's life. There is nothing I love more than helping people reach their goals.

My heart fills with joy when I see the smile on someone's face after their fitness dreams become a reality. I work with everyone from older women with extreme weight problems to special needs bodybuilders.

I have found my calling in life and that is to help as many people either through inspiring them when I compete on stage, being a mentor at FAME fitness camps, or one on one lifestyle coaching. I could not imagine doing any thing else.

# SECTION TWO
# RECIPES

# Meaty Meals

## seafood, poultry, beef

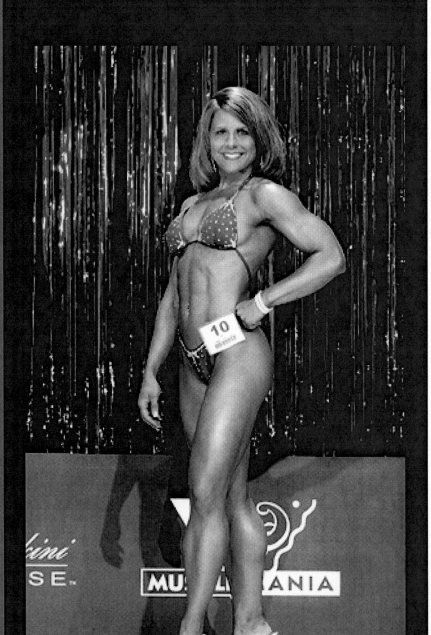

# BodyArtist

## Kim Asbury

Office Administrator and Group Fitness Instructor
Team Savage Fitness Competitor

Photo by: Gordon J Smith

It has taken a few years for me to realize that training as a fitness competitor isn't 12 weeks out from the show and then let it all drop off after the show is over.

Eating isn't about entertainment its about fueling your body so it can function properly.

I decided that I want to live a healthy life style. That doesn't mean only eating chicken and broccoli. It means finding healthy foods that you like and combining them with other foods that compliment them.

I love that the BodyArt meals are only one or two servings. They are easy to prepare and taste great.

Fitness has always been a part of my life and will continue to be a part as long as I am able. Nothing is more fulfilling or satisfying then walking out of the gym knowing that I just completed a work out and I feel great. And even more so, walking onto a stage and know that all the hard work I've done has paid off, regardless of the placing I receive.

# What to do with:
# SEAFOOD

## Tuna
(canned in water)

## White Fish
(mostly fresh Cod)

## Shrimp
(big fat ones)

# ◖ BAKED PEPPER (cheesy seafood)
*Servings: 1*
*Per serving: 214 cal, 39g Protein, 7g Carbohydrate, 3g Fat, 2g Fiber*

1 green or red bell pepper (sliced in half and cleaned)

Mix together:

  4oz (approx. 1 cup) of your favorite seafood
  (tuna, cod, sole, shrimp, or lobster)
  1 tablespoon non fat cottage cheese
  1 tablespoon non fat mayo
  1 tablespoon low fat sharp cheddar (shredded)
  2 tablespoons diced onion
  1 dash of cayenne pepper

With care, fill the pepper halves with the mixture.
Broil in toaster oven 5-7 minutes.

# ❨ COD STIR-FRY (fennel cabbage curry)

*Servings: 1*
*Per serving: 205 cal, 30g Protein, 12g Carbohydrate, 3.5g Fat, 5g Fiber*

With care, add the followiing in a deep-dish pan on medium heat:

    5 oz of raw cod (sliced)
    1 cup of water

Cover and let cook about 5 minutes.
Lower heat and toss in the following:

    1 clove or garlic (sliced) or garlic powder
    1 teaspoon oil of your choice
    2 cups shredded cabbage
    1 handful of button mushrooms (sliced)
    1 pinch of fennel powder
    1 pinch of curry powder
    1 squeeze of fresh lemon or lime

Balance on one foot and stir for a minute or two.

# ☀ CREAMED PEAS

*Servings: 2*
*Per serving: 217 cal, 24g Protein, 24g Carbohydrate, 2.5g Fat, 4.5g Fiber*


Mash together:

    1 can of tuna or 4.5oz cooked cod
    3 oz or ½ fist sized cooked potato or yam
    ¼ cup non fat plain yogurt
    1 teaspoon oil of your choice
    pinch of black pepper

Balance on one foot and stir in the following.

    1 cup peas
    1 tablespoon sharp low fat cheddar or nutritional yeast

Eat cold or warm.

# ✳☉ FISH & CHIPS

*Servings: 1*
*Per serving: 389 cal, 45g Protein, 46g Carbohydrate, 1.2g Fat, 5g Fiber*

Slice thin discs from 1 small (4oz) potato or yam
Place them on a sprayed cookie sheet leaving enough room for
the fish.  Lightly spray/spritz with oil spray.

### get out 3 plates to dress your fish

*PLATE #1*
  2 tablespoons oat flour (grind your oats in a coffee grinder)

PLATE #2 *combine the following:*
  2 tablespoons cornmeal
  pinch lemon pepper
  pinch basil
  pinch of cayenne pepper

PLATE #3
  1-2 egg whites (beat until frothy)

**Slice** 5 oz raw cod fillets into bite size pieces

**Dip** one side of fish in plate #1, shake off excess.

**Dip** other side of fish into plate #3, then plate #2.

**Place** fish on the cookie sheet cornmeal side up.

Bake at 450 degrees for 6 - 12 minutes or until fish flakes easily
with a fork.  Option: Squeeze of fresh lemon.

#  FISH CHOWDER FOR ONE

*Servings: 1*
*Per serving: 346 cal, 43g Protein, 41g Carbohydrate, 0.2g Fat, 0.8g Fiber*

With care, combine the following ingredients in a soup pot:

   1 cup of mixed seafood (cod, shrimp, crab, lobster, scallop)
   4 oz cooked potato (dice small)
   ¼ cup of chopped onion
   2 shakes black pepper
   1 cup skim or soy milk
   ½ handful of fresh cilantro chopped (optional)

Heat and Stir.

In a jar, shake 1-2 teaspoons cornstarch, ¼ cup cold water. While you're there, shake your hips too!

Just before the soup comes to a boil, pour in the cornstarch/water mixture and continue to stir.

Keep heating and stirring until it is thickened.

If it becomes too thick, just add a little water.  If not thick enough, add more cornstarch/water mixture.

HINT
Also good when add 1/8 cup of coconut milk. This will add a few extra calories and fat grams.

# ☀ FISH SANDWICH - BUT NO BREAD
*Servings: 1*
*Per serving: 295 cal, 35g Protein, 26g Carbohydrate, 4.4g Fat, 2g Fiber*

Balance on one foot and stir the following ingredients in a bowl.

   1 can of tuna or 5oz cooked white fish
   ½ cup cooked rice
   1 tablespoon nonfat mayo
   ¼ medium cucumber (diced)
   1 pinch dillweed

# ( FOUNDATION COLORS - COD DISH

*Servings: 1*
*Per serving: 290 cal, 37g Protein, 28g Carbohydrate, 4.2g Fat, 5g Fiber*

Combine the following in a deep fry pan.
Cover and let cook about 5 minutes on med/high.

　　5 oz white fish fillet
　　1-2 cloves of garlic (sliced or diced)
　　¼ small onion (chopped)
　　1 cup of water

With care, add the following to the pan and keep stirring for a couple more minutes.

　　½ cup corn kernels
　　1 medium tomato (chopped)
　　½ orange bell pepper (chopped)
　　1 teaspoon oil
　　option: pinch of fresh basil or cliantro

When the smell starts to tickle your taste buds, its done!

# ☀🚗 HARDCORE GYPSY SPECIAL

*Servings: 2*
*Per serving: 216 cal, 21g Protein, 23g Carbohydrate, 3.3g Fat, 6g Fiber*

With care, stir the following ingredients in a bowl and eat!

- 1 can of tuna drained (canned in water)
- 1 small bag (1 cup) frozen corn, peas, carrots, green beans
- 1 tablespoon raisins
- 1 handful of organic unsalted corn chips (crushed)

All of these ingredients can be found at the grocery store and combined together in a tupperware at a picinc table or the store cafe.

# 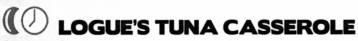 LOGUE'S TUNA CASSEROLE

*Servings: 8*
*Per serving: 150 cal, 27g Protein, 8g Carbohydrate, 0.3g Fat, 3.3g Fiber*
*Thanks to: Donna & Brian Logue*

With care, boil 20 oz California Mix until soft and mash.

Add the following ingredients, mix and press into casserole dish
sprayed with nonstick cooking spray:

    6, 4 oz cans of tuna
    4 egg whites or ½ cup egg beaters
    ½ cup chopped onions
    ½ cup sliced celery
    1 oz oatmeal
    mrs. dash
    ½ teaspoon pepper
    1 tablespoon lemon juice

Bake in oven at 350 for approximately 45 minutes.
Casserole will be firm to touch.

# ☀☉ SCALLOPED POTATOES

*Servings: 3*
*Per serving: 248 cal, 25g Protein, 31g Carbohydrate, 2.5g Fat, 0.8g Fiber*

With care, arrange the following in layers on the bottom of a non stick cassorole dish:

> 12 oz or 3 small potatoes (peel and slice into thin discs)
> ½ medium Onion (sliced)

Mix the following ingredients in a bowl and then pour it over top the potatoes and onions:

> 2 cans of tuna or 30 oz fresh white fish fillet
> 2-3 cloves garlic (sliced)
> ½ cup nonfat milk
> 1 tablespoon oil of your choice
> 1 tablespoon molly mcbutter or butter buds
> 1 pinch black pepper

Bake in oven at 350 degrees for 60 to 75 minutes or until the potatoes are browned.

# ☀ SEAFOOD CAKES

*Servings: 1*
*Per serving: 237 cal, 24g Protein, 29g Carbohydrate, 3.5g Fat, 1g Fiber*

With your hands, smoosh the following together in a bowl, then form into small mini-patties.

½ cup of seafood (cod, sole, crab, lobster, shrimp, or tuna)
1 egg white
4 oz potato or yam (mashed) or roughly one fist size
½ long green onion (chopped)
pinch of fresh parsley
dash cayenne pepper
splash of lemon juice
1 teaspoon oil of your choice

Gently place the patties in a pan on medium heat. Wait a couple minutes and flip so that they are browned on both sides.

> TIP
> The combinations here can be quite creative.
> Get playful. Try different seafoods and variety of spices.

# SHRIMP SERIES

## ◖ A: spicy shrimp

*Servings: 1*
*Per serving: 227 cal, 26g Protein, 21g Carbohydrate, 4g Fat, 7g Fiber*

With care, combine the following in a pan on medium heat:

  4 oz cooked large shrimp
  1 teaspoon oil of your choice
  1 tablespoon vinegar
  ½ tomato (chopped) or small handful cherry tomatoes
  1 large carrot (sliced)
  slice of fresh ginger (diced)
  squeeze of fresh lemon or lime
  jalapeno or thai peppers (to your taste)

Balance on one foot and stir for a few minutes.

## ◖ B: garlic and feta shrimp

*Servings: 1*
*Per serving: 185 cal, 27g Protein, 5g Carbohydrate, 4.5g Fat, 1g Fiber*

With care, combine the following in a pan on medium heat:

  4 oz cooked large shrimp
  1 teaspoon oil of your choice
  1-3 cloves of garlic (diced)
  squeeze of fresh lemon or lime
  pinch of fresh parsley
  pinch of dried thyme
  ½ cucumber (diced)

Balance on one foot and stir for a few minutes.

Top with:

  1 tablespoon fat reduced feta cheese.

**organize to optimize**

# ☾ C: coconut herb shrimp

*Servings: 1*
*Per serving: 172 cal, 25g Protein, 5g Carbohydrate, 4.5g Fat. 2g Fiber*

With care, combine the following in a pan on medium heat:

4 oz cooked large shrimp
1 teaspoon oil of your choice
1-3 cloves of garlic (diced)
¼ cup unsweetened, reduced fat coconut milk
½ green bell pepper (sliced)
½ red bell pepper (sliced)
pinch of fresh basil
pinch of fresh cilantro
pinch of fresh parsley

Balance on one foot and stir for a few minutes.

# ✳ SIMPLE - TUNA, FIBER & PINEAPPLE

*Servings: 1*

*Per serving: 356 cal, 37.5g Protein, 44g Carbohydrate, 4.2g Fat, 9g Fiber*

With excitement for your meal, combine the following and heat:

    1 can of tuna (canned in water or fresh)
    2 cups (about 10 oz) frozen green & yellow beans
    1 teaspoon oil
    ½ cup or small jar basil & oregano tomato sauce
    ½ cup of crushed pineapple

# ☾ STACY'S QUICK TUNA MIRACLE

*Servings: 1*
*Per serving: 229 cal, 25g Protein, 22g Carbohydrate, 3.5g Fat, 8g Fiber*

With care, mix it all together in your favorite bowl…done!

½ can tuna (or 3oz white fish)
1 cup of mixed veggies (peas, corn, carrots)
1 tablespoon low fat mayo

# ☀ SUPER FAST FISH WRAP

*Servings: 1*
*Per serving: 297 cal, 27.5g Protein, 31g Carbohydrate, 7g Fat, 5g Fiber*

With care and a big smile (you know this takes no time to make!), combine the following in a bowl:

½ can of tuna or 3 oz cooked white fish
2 tablespoons of salsa
1 tablespoon fat free cream cheese

Scoop the mixture down the middle of a warmed tortilla.
Option: Add some salad greens and onions to the mixture.

## TORTILLA FOLDING INSTRUCTIONS

step 1:
Fold one end of the tortilla away from you and tuck the edge under the mound of food.

step 2:
Wrap your fingers under the tucked edge and scrape the food toward you using the tucked edge. Firmly pack the food into a log shape that sits in the tortilla fold.

step 3:
Fold in the ends and roll the food-packed log away from you until it is fully wraped in the whole tortilla.

# ( STUFFED MUSHROOMS

*Servings: 1*
*Per serving: 179 cal, 22g Protein, 15g Carbohydrate, 4.4g Fat, 3g Fiber*
*Thanks to Richard Erno*

With care, combine the following in a bowl:

½ cup of seafood (your choice of one or combination of many)
1 tablespoon fat reduced mayo
¼ cucumber (diced)
1 green onion (scallion) (diced)
pinch of your favorite spice
*(dill, basil, sage, rosemary, thyme, tarragon, parsley, or coriander)*

Pull the stems out of 6-8 large button mushrooms. There should be a natural hole in the cap to stuff the filling mixture.

Chop the mushroom stems and add them to the rest of the ingredients to form your filling - or save them in the fridge for a late-night omlette filler.

Stuff the mushroom caps as full as you can. Place them on a cookie sheet or in a muffin tray.

Broil for about 5-8 minutes.

TIP
Allow them to cool a little before eating. The juices are hot.

Option:
Top with a tablespoon of sharp cheddar and add a couple grams of fat.

These are so fun to share - a great snack for your fitness friends!

# ☀ **TANGY WRAP**

*Servings: 1*
*Per serving: 295 cal, 23g Protein, 29g Carbohydrate, 10.5g Fat, 6g Fiber*

With some salsa music in the background, mix the following in a bowl (be sure to shake your bootie):

½ can of tuna or 3oz cooked white fish
1 tablespoon reduced fat mayo or nonfat plain yogurt
1 teaspoon relish or one chopped dill pickle
½ teaspoon horseradish

Warm 1 large whole wheat or spinach tortilla.

Scoop the filling down the middle of the tortilla and add a handful of salad greens.

## TORTILLA FOLDING INSTRUCTIONS

step 1:
Fold one end of the tortilla away from you and tuck the edge under the mound of food.

step 2:
Wrap your fingers under the tucked edge and scrape the food toward you using the tucked edge. Firmly pack the food into a log shape that sits in the tortilla fold.

step 3:
Fold in the ends and roll the food-packed log away from you until it is fully wraped in the whole tortilla.

# ☀ TANYA'S TUNA SANDWICH

Servings: 1
Per serving: 322 cal, 26g Protein, 34g Carbohydrate, 9.6g Fat, 10g Fiber

With care, mix the following in a bowl:

½ can of tuna (canned in water or fresh)
½ small or ¼ medium avacado
1 long green onion or scallion (chopped)

Spread the mixture onto 2 slices sprouted/grainy bread.

> TIP
> Grill it in a lightly misted pan or in a sandwich grill and cut into triangles. Share as snacks for guests or kids.

Option: Dip the outside of the sandwich in egg white and then grill it! This also adds a couple more grams of protein to your meal.

# ☾ THAI COD WITH RED CURRY

*Servings: 1*
*Per serving: 211 cal, 29g Protein, 12g Carbohydrate, 4.5g Fat, 6g Fiber*

With care, pour the following into a medium-heat pan.

> ¼ cup light unsweetened coconut milk
> 1 toothpick end of red curry paste (this stuff is powerful)
> 1-2 pinches of chopped fresh coriander or basil
> 1-2 pinch of preferred sweetener

Balance on one foot and stir for a couple minutes.
Then add the following.

> 4oz cod fillet
> 1 medium zuchinni (sliced)
> ½ red bell pepper (sliced)

Balance on the other foot and stire for another minute or two.
Then add the following:

> 2 big handfuls of baby spinach

Top with a squeeze of fresh lime/lemon.

# ☀ THAI SURPRISE

*Servings: 1*
*Per serving: 412 cal, 35g Protein, 59g Carbohydrate, 5g Fat, 12g Fiber*
without rice:
*Per serving: 303 cal, 33g Protein, 36g Carbohydrate, 4g Fat, 10g Fiber*
*Thanks to Richard Erno*


With care, heat your pan or wok to medium.  Add about 1 cup of water and 5 oz of raw cod (sliced or not). Cover and let cook about 5 minutes.

Balance on one foot and stir in the following:

    1 teaspoons oil of your choice
    1 medium (6 oz) carrot (sliced)
    ½ cucumber (chopped)
    3 button mushrooms (sliced)
    1 cup cut frozen green beans
    1 splash of low sodium soy sauce or braggs liquid aminos
    1 pinch of dill
    1 pinch of thai spice
    ½ cup cooked rice

Cook and stir for another 5 minutes or so.

# ◖ T 'n' T TUNA AND TURNIPS

*Servings: 1*

*Per serving: 185 cal, 19g Protein, 20g Carbohydrate, 3.3g Fat, 8g Fiber*


½ can of tuna or 3 oz cooked white fish

16 oz or 2 ½ cups of cooked turnip cut in cubes or mashed

1 teaspoon oil of your choice

1 dash of onion powder

optional dash of molly mcbutter or butter buds


With care, MASH everything together. Heat when you want to eat!

# 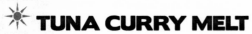 TUNA CURRY MELT

*Servings: 1*
*Per serving: 305 cal, 30g Protein, 30g Carbohydrate, 7g Fat, 6g Fiber*

With some Janis Joplin in the background, mix the following:

  ½ can of tuna (canned in water or fresh)
  1 tablespoon fat reduced mayo
  1 good pinch of curry (experiment to your tastes)
  1 scallion (green onion) cut with scissors

Scoop on to:

  2 slices sprouted/grainy bread

Top with:

  2 tablespoons low fat sharp cheddar

Grill your lovely sandwich with a light mist of spray oil.

TIP
Make it "open-face", scooping the filling on top of each
of the pieces of bread, top with cheddar and place on a
cookie sheet in the oven on broil for a few minutes.
rill it in a lightly misted pan or in a sandwich grill and cut
into triangles. Share as snacks for guests or kids.

**every baby step matters**

# ◖ TUNA HELPER - HOME MADE

*Servings: 1*
*Per serving: 327 cal, 32g Protein, 38g Carbohydrate, 3.3g Fat, 8.5g Fiber*

With care, HEAT a non stick deep-dish pan to medium.
Toss in the following and stir them around:

- ¼ small onion (diced)
- 1-2 cloves of garlic (sliced or minced)
- 1 teaspoon oil of your choice

Balance on one foot and stir in the following.

- ½ can of tuna or 3 oz cooked white fish
- 1 cup of frozen or fresh peas
- 1 cup skim milk or nonfat soy milk
- 1 pinch fresh basil
- 1 dash cayenne pepper

Just before it looks like it is going to boil, stir in the following:

- 1 tablespoon cornstarch (shake in jar with 1/8 cup cold water)

Lower the heat and simmer.
Balance on the other foot and gently stir.

In 1-2 minutes you should notice it beginning to thicken.

OPTION: top with a 2 tablespoons of grated sharp cheddar (add 4 grams of fat)

# ( VEGGIES & FISH DIP

*Servings: 1*
*Per serving: 265 cal, 23g Protein, 42g Carbohydrate, 1g Fat, 4g Fiber*

With care, blend a thick scooping-style dip from the following:

½ can of tuna or 3 oz cooked white fish
½ small potato or 3oz (cooked)
1 teaspoon horseradish
¼ cup plain nonfat yogurt
1 long green onion or scallion (chopped)
fresh lemon squeeze

Wash a variety of the following:

1 ½ cups fresh raw veggies
(carrots, mushrooms, celery, brocolli, etc.)

Scoop the dip onto the veggies and enjoy!

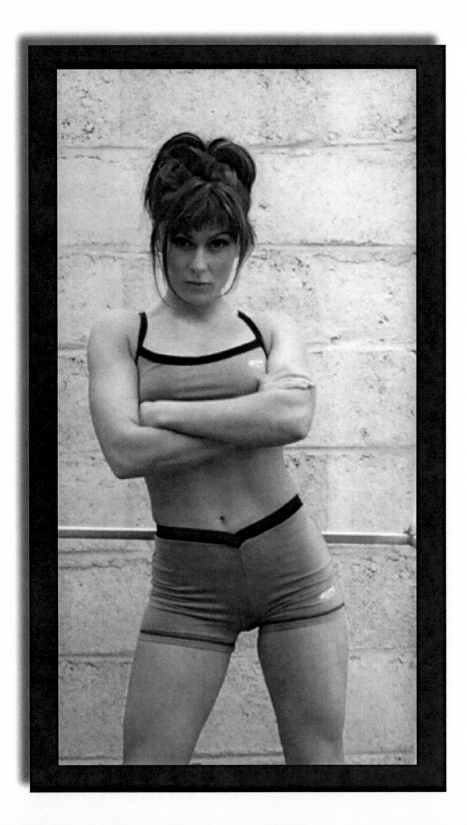

# BodyArtist

## Michele Theoret

Owner: The Power Center
Yoga, Fitness, Body Transformation
www.getempowerednow.ca

My practice is not always easy but it is always the truth, a mirror into my life, a direct reflection of where I am at in the present moment.

In a difficult pose when I am struggling with every bone of my being to hold on, I go inside with my breath and become aware of my resistance. I feel myself at war just trying to survive and win at all costs, and then with a deep exhale I let it go. No judgment.

Being a wife, mother, daughter, sister and friend is no different, there are moments when we begin to lose control; however my practice has given me that option of just simply breathing and being fully present to my thoughts and actions. Yoga creates space for conciousness and this will change your life and the world around you.

The Truth is there is no magic pill or perfect exercise. Find something that feeds both your body and your soul, continue to be honest with yourself and commit. I sincerely believe that anybody can accomplish anything they dream, if the intention and willingness is there.

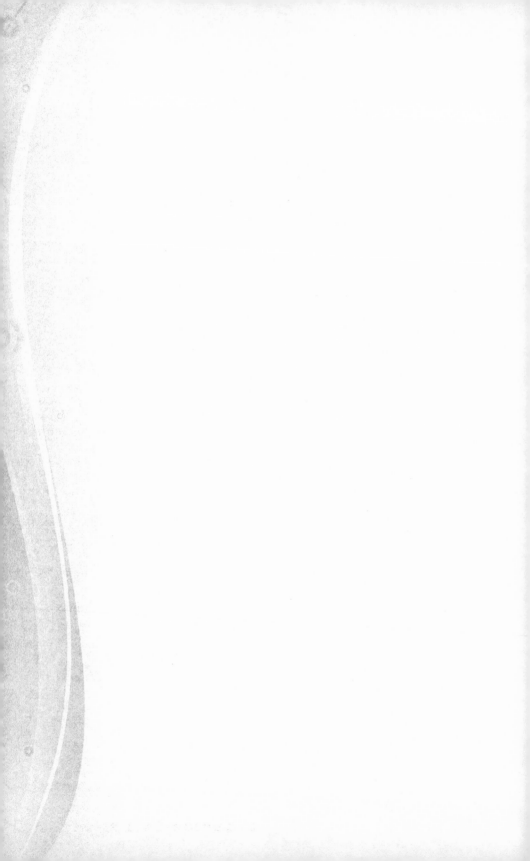

# What to do with:
# POULTRY

## Chicken
(breast meat)

## Turkey
(breast meat)

# ( BASIC CHICKEN STIR-FRY

*Servings: 1*
*Per serving: 270 cal, 33g Protein, 22g Carbohydrate,  6.5g Fat, 8g Fiber*

With care, combine all ingredients into a deep-dish pan on medium heat (may have to add a splash of water):

  1 small (3oz)cooked chicken breast half(sliced or diced)
  10 oz (2-3 big handfuls) mixed oriental or fibrous veggies
  1 clove fresh garlic (or teaspoon of pre-minced or powdered)
  1 slice fresh ginger root (minced/grated)
  1 tablespoon rice vinegar
  1 pinch preferred sweetener
  1 squeeze of fresh lemon or lime

Cover for a few minutes.
Lower heat and stir in:

  1 teaspoon oil

Stir for a minute to let the flavors blend.

*If chicken is uncooked then put the chicken in first until almost done and then add everything else.*

# ☀ CANDY SWEET POTATO MASH

*Servings: 1*
*Per serving: 264 cal, 29.5g Protein, 28g Carbohydrate, 3g Fat, 6.5g Fiber*

Whip the following ingredients with a hand-blender until fluffy:

   4 oz or 1 small cooked sweet potato or yam (cubed)
   1 cup cooked rutabaga or turnip(cubed)
   2 drops maple extract
   1 pinch cinnamon
   1 pinch preferred sweetener
   1 tablespoon water

Stir in 1 small (3oz)cooked chicken breast half(sliced or diced).

#  CHICKEN FRIED RICE IN SECONDS

*Servings: 1*
*Per serving: 312 cal, 38.5g Protein, 28.5g Carbohydrate, 4g Fat, 4g Fiber*

Toss the following ingredients into a deep dish pan or wok:

1 small (3oz)cooked chicken breast half(diced small)
½ cup cooked brown rice
½ stalk celery (chopped)
¼ cup frozen or fresh peas
1 egg or 2 egg whites
1/3 cup water
1 dash black pepper
1 dash low sodium chinese spice (optional)
squirt of bragg's amino acids
squeeze of fresh lemon or lime

Stir and cover for a few minutes.

NOTE
If the chicken is not pre-cooked, throw it in the pan first with
a little water to steam. When it is almost cooked, add the
rest of the ingredients into a pan on med.-high heat.

If the chicken is pre-cooked, then just throw everything in
all at once.

# ✳ CHICKEN FRY 'KIYOMI' STYLE

*Servings: 1*
*Per serving: 289 calo, 31g Protein, 31g Carbohydrate, 4g Fat, 5g Fiber*
*Thanks to Kiyomi Shigemi*

Toss the following ingredients into a deep dish pan or wok:

> 1 small (3oz)cooked chicken breast half(diced small)5 oz or 1-2 cups fresh or frozen broccoli (chopped)
> ½ cup brown rice
> 1 tablespoon red wine vinegar
> 1 teaspoon curry powder
> 1 teaspoon ginger
> ½ teaspoon paprika

If the chicken is not pre-cooked, throw it in the pan first with a little water to steam. When it is almost cooked, (with care) add the rest of the ingredients into a pan on med.-high heat. If the chicken is pre-cooked, then just throw everything in all at once.

#  CHICKEN MUSHROOM RICE

*Servings: 1*
*Per serving: 344 cal, 32g Protein, 37.5g Carbohydrate, 6.7g Fat, 4g Fiber*
*Thanks to Steven Sowinski*

With care, combine the following in a heated pot . Balance on one foot and stir until warmed.  Add any desired seasonings.

    1 small (3oz)cooked chicken breast half(sliced or diced)
    ½ cup cooked rice
    ¼ cup water
    ½ can low fat mushroom soup
    handful of button mushrooms
    shallots (chopped)

NOTE
If you don't have rice cooked, combine one part rice with one part water, add the soup, mishrooms and shallots - bring to a boil for 5 minutes. Cover and let sit for 15 minutes. Add chicken.

This recipe also works well with seafood and beef.

# ☀ CHICKEN PIZZA MUSH

*Servings: 1*
*Per serving: 329 cal, 35g Protein, 37g Carbohydrate, 4.5g Fat, 5g Fiber*

With care, toss a handful of sliced onions into a medium heat non-stick pan with a little bit of water.

Once the onions are softened, mix the following and add to the pan.

> 2 tablespoons tomato paste
> 3 tablespoons water
> 1 pinch basil
> 1 pinch oregano
> 1 pinch garlic powder (or fresh garlic)

Add the following:

> 1 small (3oz)cooked chicken breast half(diced small)
> ½ cup cooked rice
> ¼ cup pineapple chunks or tidbits

Balance on one foot and stir until it is heated how you like it. (I like my rice a little crispy!)

Top with 2 tablespoons low fat cottage cheese.

# ☪ CHICKEN VEGGIE GOULASH

*Servings: 2*
*Per serving: 234cal, 33g Protein, 19g Carbohydrate, 4g Fat, 6.5g Fiber*
*Thanks to Denise Knorr*

In a pot, combine the following:

    1 handful of mushrooms, whole
    1 med. green bell pepper (diced)…great vitamin c source!
    1 med. yellow bell pepper (diced)
    ½ small onion (diced)
    2 handfuls or 6 oz of cauliflower

With care, mix the following and add to the pot.

    2 tablespoons tomato paste
    2 dashes black pepper
    2 dashes italian ms. dash
    1 dash crushed chili peppers
    2 dashes oregano
    optional fresh basil
    1 teaspoon minced garlic (or couple fresh cloves)

Cover and on med-high heat until you are happy with the texture of the veggies.

Stir in 2 diced small cooked chicken breast halves (6oz).

Top with squeeze from fresh lime and 1 cup alfalfa sprouts

NOTE
If your chicken is not pre-cooked, add it in at the beginning and cook until almost done, then add everything else.

**every baby step matters**

# ☀ CITRUS STIR-FRY

*Servings: 1*
*Per serving: 299 cal, 32g Protein, 34g Carbohydrate 4g Fat, 6g Fiber*
*Thanks to Rhonda Lent*


With care, toss the following into a medium heated pan.

   1 small (3oz)cooked chicken breast half(diced)
   1 large handful or 5 oz of oriental vegetable mix
   ¼ cup of real lemon juice or squeeze one real lemon
   3 shakes of lemon pepper

Add about ½ cup water. Cover until the veggies are warm.

Pour the mixture over ½ cup cooked rice.

#  CREAMED CORN MASH POTATO

*Servings: 1*
*Per serving: 333 cal, 33g Protein, 43g Carbohydrate, 5g Fat, 3g Fiber*

With care, combine the following in a container. HEAT when you are ready to eat!

  1 small (3oz)cooked chicken breast half(diced)
  1 sm or 3oz potato or yam (mashed or baked)
  ½ cup frozen corn
  1 tablespoon non-fat plain yogurt
  ¼ med. green bell pepper
  1 dash onion powder
  1 dash chili powder

# ☾☀ EASY CHEESY MIXED VEG

*Servings: 1*
*Per serving: 265 cal, 37g Protein, 18g Carbohydrate, 3.5g Fat,  6g Fiber*

With care and a big smile of joy, cause it's so easy, toss the following into a non-stick pan on med heat.

    1 small (3oz)cooked chicken breast half(pull into chunks or not)
    1cup frozen peas, carrots, corn, and green beans
    2 tablespoons non fat cottage cheese
    optional spices ( i like taco spice)

Stir and cover for a few minutes until the veggies thaw and the cheese starts to melt.

TIP
Toss it all into a container and take it to go. The frozen veggies will keep the chicken cool until its time to eat!

# ☀ FAJITA CHICKEN WRAP

*Servings: 1*
*Per serving: 362 cal, 35g Protein, 34g Carbohydrate 12g Fat, 7g Fiber*

With care, combine the following in a medium-heat pan.

  1 small (3oz)cooked chicken breast halfsliced)
  few slices of purple onion
  1 med red, yellow, or green bell pepper (sliced)
  1-2 cloves of garlic (cut or crushed)
  1 dash dried chili peppers
  1 pinch chili powder
  squeeze of fresh lime

Heat and stir until your veggies are the way you like them.

Warm a tortilla (i like spinach or tomato flavor) and spread on it:

  1 tablespoon non-fat sour cream
  1 tablespoon salsa

Pour the pan mixture down the middle of the tortilla (it should be thick, not runny).

## TORTILLA FOLDING INSTRUCTIONS

step 1:
Fold one end of the tortilla away from you and tuck the edge under the mound of food.

step 2:
Wrap your fingers under the tucked edge and scrape the food toward you using the tucked edge. Firmly pack the food into a log shape that sits in the tortilla fold.

step 3:
Fold in the ends and roll the food-packed log away from you until it is fully wraped in the whole tortilla.

**every baby step matters**

# ☾ GREEN BEANS & MUSHROOMS

*Servings: 1*
*Per serving: 267 cal, 32g Protein, 22g Carbohydrate, 6.6g Fat, 5g Fiber*

With care, combine the following in a medium-heat pan.

   1 small (3oz)cooked chicken breast half(diced)
   2 cups or 10 oz of green beans
   1 handful or about 4 fresh mushrooms (sliced)
   1-2 slices of purple onion

Balance on one foot and stir.
Cover and let cook until everything is warm.
Stir in:

   1 teaspoon oil

# ☀ HASH BROWN PATTY

*Servings: 1*
*Per serving: 302 cal, 38g Protein, 31g Carbohydrate, 4g Fat. 2g Fiber*

In your favorite bowl, mix the following and then form it into a pattie with your hands.

    1 small (3oz)cooked chicken breast half(diced or shredded)
    1 small or 3oz potato or yam (mashed or baked and smooshed)
    ¼ cup corn
    2 egg whites or ¼ cup egg beaters
    ½ green onion (snipped) or dry chives
    1 dash cayenne pepper
    1 dash paprika
    1 dash garlic powder (or real garlic)

Gently place the pattie into med-hot pan with cooking spray.

Flip so both sides are browned…takes about 5 minutes.

Don't make the patty too thick making the middle doughy.

# ☀ HEAVENLY MASHED POTATOES

*Servings: 1*
*Per serving: 275 cal, 31g Protein, 31g Carbohydrate, 3g Fat, 1g Fiber*

With care, combine the following in a container to heat later, or in a pot on the stove.

- 1 small (3oz)cooked chicken breast half(pull into chunks)
- 1 med. or 4oz potato or yam (mashed or baked and smooshed)
- 1 teaspoon defatted, low-sodium chicken broth powder
- 1 garlic clove (minced)
- 1 pinch pepper

TIP
If you heat it in a skillet on the stove with a little oil or spray, you can get the potatoes crispy.

**organize to optimize**

# ☾ HOT GARLIC CHICKEN SALAD

*Servings: 1*
*Per serving: 197 cal, 31g Protein, 12g Carbohydrate, 3g Fat, 4g Fiber*

Playfully toss the following into a medium-heat pan with a splash of water.

    1 small (3oz) cooked chicken breast half(sliced)
    few slices of onion
    1-3 cloves of garlic (minced)

Balance on one foot and stir for a few minutes until the garlic is softened, or if the chicken is not pre-cooked...it takes about 10 minutes to cook up raw chicken chunks - so make sure to switch the leg you are  balancing on.

In a jar, shake the following to make a dressing.
While you're there, shake your hips too!

    few splashes of balsamic vinegar
    squeeze of fresh lemon

Pour the dressing over 3 big handfuls (3-4 cups) of mixed greens (darker the better!).

Top with the warm chicken mixture and 2-3 sliced cherry tomatoes.

**every baby step matters**

# ☀ HOT QUICKY WRAP

*Servings: 1*
*Per serving: 352 cal, 35g Protein, 32g Carbohydrate, 11g Fat. 6g Fiber*

With care, warm the following in a pan.

　　1 small (3oz)cooked chicken breast half(sliced or diced or not)
　　splashes of hot sauce (to your taste)

Smear 1 tablespoon non-fat sour cream down the middle of a
warmed tortilla and top with handful of mixed salad greens and
perhaps a squeeze of fresh lime.

## TORTILLA FOLDING INSTRUCTIONS

step 1:
Fold one end of the tortilla away from you and tuck the edge under
the mound of food.

step 2:
Wrap your fingers under the tucked edge and scrape the food
toward you using the tucked edge. Firmly pack the food into a log
shape that sits in the tortilla fold.

step 3:
Fold in the ends and roll the food-packed log away from you until it
is fully wraped in the whole tortilla.

# 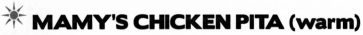 MAMY'S CHICKEN PITA (warm)

*Servings: 1*
*Per serving: 317 cal, 39g Protein, 25g Carbohydrate 8g Fat, 3g Fiber*

With care, make a pocket from ½ large whole wheat pita and fill it
with the following mixture:

    1 small (3oz)cooked chicken breast half (diced or not)
    2 tablespoons nonfat cottage cheese
    1/8 cup low fat cheddar shredded
    3 tomato slices
    squirt of dijon mustard

Heat in toaster oven for 5 minutes.

Add 1 handful of mixed salad greens and enjoy.

#  MOTO CHICKEN (my brothers meal)

*Servings: 1*

*Per serving: 324 cal, 31g Protein, 35g Carbohydrate, 7g Fat, 3g Fiber*

With care and dreams of soaring across the sky off a motocross jump, toss the following into a medium-heat pan.

1 small (3oz)cooked chicken breast half (pull into chunks or not)
1 medium potato or yam (4 oz) mashed, baked or boiled
½ med. green bell pepper (sliced)
large handful or 4 med. mushrooms (sliced)
1 long green onion or scallion (snipped)
1 teaspoon coconut, hemp, or olive oil
pinch of black pepper

Balance on one foot and stir for a few minutes. If my brother can cook…anyone can!

> NOTE
> Some people simply don't have the taste for veggies right now. My little brother is a motocross daredevil and won't eat anything green except bell peppers. The only veggies he will eat are listed in this recipe. Seriously!

# ☀ "NO ROLL" CHICK CABBAGE ROLL

*Servings: 1*
*Per serving: 300 cal, 33g Protein, 35g Carbohydrate, 4g Fat, 9g Fiber*

For a couple minutes, boil 2 cups cabbage (cut or shredded) - not long, just enough to slightly soften.

Mix the following in a bowl and then stir it into the cabbage pot (drain the water first).

 1 small (3oz)cooked chicken breast half (sliced or diced)
 ¼ sm. onion (chopped)
 ½ med. tomato (diced)
 2 tablespoons tomato paste
 1 pinch preferred sweetener
 ¼ cup water
 1 squirt mustard
 1 dash black pepper
 1 dash garlic powder
 1 dash oregano
 1/3 cup cooked brown rice
 1 splash rice vinegar

Let simmer for a couple of minutes.

TIP
I usually make 5 times the amount in a big pot, then separate it into 5 equal containers.

# ☀ ☾ 'NO BUN' CHICKEN BURGER

*Servings: 1*
*Per serving: 223 cal, 37g Protein, 12g Carbohydrate, 4g Fat, 4g Fiber*
*Thanks to Lorriane Birch*

Mix the following together with your hands and then form into 1-2 small patties.

    3oz cooked chicken breast half(ground)
    1 egg or 2 egg whites
    ¼ cup rolled oats
    1 long green onion (snipped)
    ¼ med. red bell pepper (chopped)
    ¼ med. zucchini (grated)
    1 tablespoon tomato paste
    1 garlic clove (minced)
    2 dashes black pepper

Place the patty in non-stick pan on on medium heat.

Takes about 10 minutes to cook all the way through (flip ½ way).

You can also use a double sided sandwich grill for this recipe.

# ☾ PORTABELLO CHICKEN PIZZA

*Servings: 1*
*Per serving: 270 cal, 38g Protein, 22g Carbohydrate, 5.5g Fat, 6g Fiber*

With care, mix together the following.

   2 tablespoons tomato paste
   little water (until paste is a pizza sauce consistency)
   dash each of basil, oregano, fennel
   2 cloves garlic (sliced) or add garlic powder

Spread the mixture on 2 large portabello mushroom caps

Top with:

   1 small (3oz)cooked chicken breast half (sliced or diced)
   1/8 cup chopped onion
   ¼ medium green bell pepper (diced)
   1-2 sliced black olives (optional)
   2 tablespoons low fat cheddar cheese (shredded)

Broil in oven about 5-10 minutes

# ☾☀ QUICK CHICKEN FINGERS

*Servings: 1*
*Per serving: 339 cal, 41g Protein, 23g Carbohydrate, 8g Fat, 6g Fiber*

Do a little song and dance as you...

Slice into strips:

   4oz cooked or raw chicken breast half

Dip into:

   2 egg whites or 1 whole egg

Then dip into mixture of:

   ¼ cup oat bran
   1 pinch cayenne pepper
   1 pinch garlic powder

Place the strips into a medium-heat pan with 1 teaspoon oil.
If you have any egg mixture left over, pour that in too!
Flip and then add the following to the pan.

   ½ med green bell pepper (sliced)
   ½ med onion (sliced)

Cover and cook until your happy with the creation.

NOTE
If you are using raw chicken, make sure there is no pink
color left in the middle of the meat.

# ❨ THAI CHICKEN

*Servings: 2*
*Per serving: 357 cal, 34g Protein, 29g Carbohydrate, 12g Fat, 10g Fiber*

With care, toss the following in a medium-heat pan.

   1 small (3oz)cooked chicken breast half(sliced or diced)
   dash garlic powder
   dash curry powder
   ¼ cup onion (sliced)
   splash of sodium reduced soy sauce

Balance on one foot and stir for a couple minutes.
Then add the following.

   ½ red pepper (sliced)
   ½ cup sliced chestnuts
   1 cup bamboo shoots
   ½ cup lite, unsweetened coconut milk
   ½ cup peas

Turn heat down to low-med.
Let simmer for a couple of minutes.
Stir occasionally.

# ☀🕐 TANDOORI CHICKEN & POTATO

*Servings: 1*
*Per serving: 349 cal, 32g Protein, 37g Carbohydrate, 9.5g Fat, 3g Fiber*

*Requires overnight marinade.*

Mix the following together in a casserole dish:

  ¾ teaspoon dijon mustard
  squeeze juice from one lemon
  1 teaspoon oil
  1/8 cup non fat plain yogurt
  couple slices fresh ginger
  1 pinch cumin
  1 pinch coriander
  1 pinch turmeric
  1 pinch chili powder (to taste)
  splash white wine

Place the following into the sauce mixture:

  1 breast or about 4 ounces raw chicken breast

Completely cover the chicken in sauce.
Put a lid on the casserole dish.
Let sit in the fridge overnight.

THE NEXT DAY...

Place the following into the dish with the chicken/sauce.

  1 medium potato or yam or about 4 ounces (cubed)

Bake for about 40 minutes at about 350-400 degrees, or put it on the barbeque.

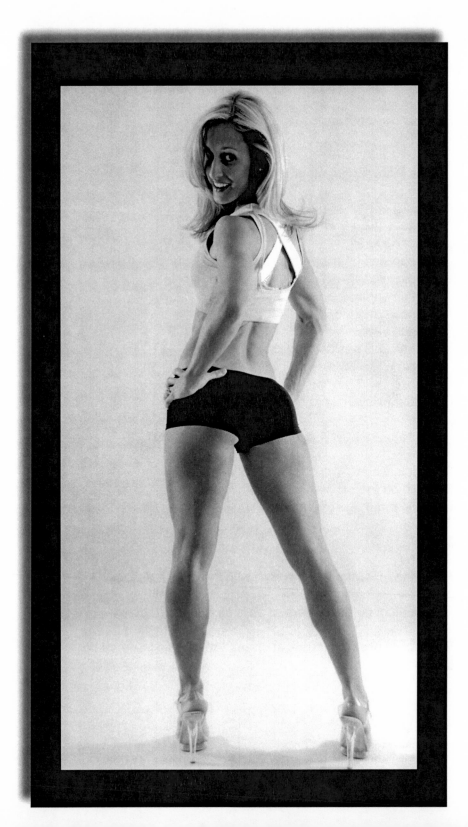

# BodyArtist

## Rachel Ibbison

Fifth Grade and Special Education Teacher
Cathy Savage Fitness Competitor
www.rachelibbison.com

Photo by: Todd Ganci

The feeling of being healthy is what motivates me everyday. In 2007 I took it to a new level of competing in fitness. The journey through this process has been such a life lesson of discipline and self fulfillment.

I have learned how important it is to stay active and eat healthy as my way of fighting the everyday struggles of life. Everyone's life can go up and down day to day. Exercise is something that gives me energy and I know exactly what types of foods my body needs to keep my energy consistent. I don't get the highs and lows like people can from eating sweets or fast foods. I eat just enough to fulfill my body, but not too much to feel completely full, and bring down my energies.

If everything in my life is not going great I know that I can still hold on to exercising and eating right. This is something that I can do for myself. The BodyArt Cookbook was actually the first book that I bought to get myself into all of this!

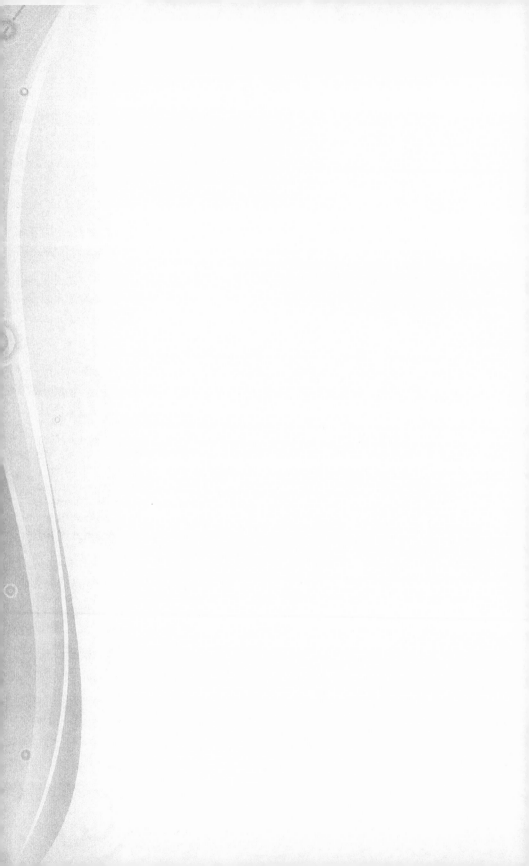

# What to do with:
# BEEF

## Lean Ground
### (sirlion or inside round)

## Steak
### (sirlion or inside round)

# BEEF BELL PEPPER HEMP RICE

*Servings: 1*
*Per serving: 337 cal, 32g Protein, 29g Carbohydrate, 10g Fat, 7g Fiber*

With care, toss the following in a medium-heat pan.

¼ med. green bell pepper (sliced)
¼ med. yellow bell pepper (sliced)
¼ med. red bell pepper
splash of water

Balance on one foot and stir until peppers are slightly softened, then toss in the following.

3 ounces of cooked lean cut of steak (sliced)
½ cup cooked brown rice
1 pinch oregano
1 tablespoon hemp hearts
squeeze of fresh lemon or lime

Balance on the other foot, continue to stir until it's all warm.

TIP
Multiply this recipe by 4 to use whole peppers at one time.

# ☾ BEEF & BROCCOLI HUNAN

*Servings: 1*
*Per serving: 233 cal, 29g Protein, 12g Carbohydrate, 7g Fat, 4g Fiber*

With care, toss the following in a medium-heat pan.

3 oz raw lean steak (cut into thin slices)
1 clove garlic (diced)
1-2 slices of fresh ginger (chopped fine)
¼ cup chopped Onion

Balance on one foot and stir for a couple minutes.
Then toss in the following.

2 cups broccoli (chopped)
¼ cup water

Balance on the other foot, turn up the heat and bring to a boil.

With care, mix the following in a bowl.

3 teaspoons cornstarch dissolved in ¼ cup water
Dash of dried red peppers or fresh spicy thai peppers
Splash of sodium reduced soy sauce
Pinch of preferred sweetener
1 teaspoon oil

Pour it into the pan and stir. watch it thicken.
If it gets too thick just add a little more water.

Let simmer for a minute or two. Enjoy.

# ☀ BEEF CHOW MEIN

*Servings: 1*
*Per serving: 257 cal, 30g Protein, 29g Carbohydrate, 2.7g Fat, 5g Fiber*

With care, toss the following in a medium-heat pan.

   3 oz raw lean steak (cut into thin slices)
   ¼ cup onions chopped

Balance on one foot and stir for a couple minutes, then add the following and cover for a couple more minutes.

   dash of black pepper
   1 stalk of celery chopped
   ¼ cup water

Add the following and bring to a low boil.

   ½ can bean sprouts drained (or equivalent fresh)

In a glass jar, shake the following. While you're there shake your hips too!

   splash of low sodium soy sauce
   pinch of preferred sweetener
   1/8 cup cold water
   2 teaspoons cornstarch

As you stir the boiling pan, pour in the jar mixture.
Continue to stir  until the sauce thickens.
Pour the contents of the pan over top of:

   ½ cup cooked rice

# ☀-⏱ BEEF PIZZA (i'm not kidding!)

*Servings: 6*
*Per serving: 229 cal, 25g Protein, 23g Carbohydrate, 4g Fat, 3g Fiber*

*option to add ¼ cup low fat mozza or cheddar cheese:*
*Per serving: 242 cal, 26.5g Protein, 23g Carbohydrate, 4.8g Fat, 3g Fiber*

## STEP ONE: Make Your Crust

With care, mix the following in a bowl and spread it on to the bottom of a square cake pan (non stick).

    2 cups of cooked short grain brown rice
    3 egg whites
    1 cup nonfat cottage cheese
    2-3 cloves of garlic (sliced)

Bake at 450 degrees for 20 minutes.

## STEP TWO: Make Your Sauce

With care, mix the following in a bowl.

    1 small can of tomato paste (plus one can full of water)
    2 teaspoons oregano
    2 teaspoons basil (try fresh)
    ½ teaspoon ground fennel (optional)
    1 pinch of crushed red peppers

Spred the sauce over your crust and top with the following.

    ½ medium green pepper (sliced)
    ½ medium onion (sliced)
    12 ounces of cooked lean cut of steak (sliced)

Bake for another 10 minutes.
Cut into 6 pieces.

You can also top with a couple tablespoons of Sharp Cheddar or some Nutritional Yeast. Add a couple grams of fat for the cheese.

This one also tastes good with Chicken instead of Beef.

# ☀ BEEF WRAP

*Servings: 1*
*Per serving: 357 cal, 33g Protein, 30g Carbohydrate, 13g Fat, 5g Fiber*

With care, toss the following in a medium-heat pan.

   3 ounces of cooked lean cut of steak (sliced)
   1-2 teaspoons chopped onion
   1 clove garlic chopped
   3 tablespoons salsa
   pinch chili powder

Warm-up:

   1 whole wheat or spinach or corn tortilla

Spread:

   1 tablespoon no-fat sour cream

Place the pan mixture down the center of the tortilla.

## TORTILLA FOLDING INSTRUCTIONS

step 1:
Fold one end of the tortilla away from you and tuck the edge under the mound of food.

step 2:
Wrap your fingers under the tucked edge and scrape the food toward you using the tucked edge. Firmly pack the food into a log shape that sits in the tortilla fold.

step 3:
Fold in the ends and roll the food-packed log away from you until it is fully wraped in the whole tortilla.

# ☀ BEEFY CREAM OF WHEAT

*Servings: 1*
*Per serving: 310 cal, 31g Protein, 35g Carbohydrate, 6.5g Fat, 1.5g Fiber*

With care, place the following in a small pot on med-high for about 5 minutes...keep stirring. Balance on one leg and then the other while you continue to stir.

   3 tablespoons cream of wheat (uncooked)
   1 cup water

Once the cereal starts to thicken, stir in the following.

   3 ounces of cooked lean beef
   1 dash black pepper
   1 tablespoon low fat sour cream

# ❰ BEEFY GREEN BEANS

*Servings: 1*
*Per serving: 279 cal, 33g Protein, 19g Carbohydrate, 8.5g Fat, 7g Fiber*

With care, toss the following into a skillet or a 'to go' container.

   3 ounces of cooked lean cut of steak (sliced)
   10 ounces (2 cups)cut green beans (fresh or frozen)
   1 tablespoon hemp seeds
   1 dash black pepper
   squeeze of fresh lemon

Balance on one foot and stir until blended and warm.

TIP
Tastes great when you cook onion into the beef.

# ☀ BEEFY 'PIZZA-LIKE' MUSH

*Servings: 1*
*Per serving: 277 cal, 33g Protein, 23g Carbohydrate, 5.5g Fat, 3g Fiber*

With care, toss the following in a medium-heat pan.

   3 ounces of cooked lean cut of steak (sliced)
   ¼ small onion (chopped)
   3 large mushrooms (sliced or chopped)
   ½ sm. to med. green pepper (sliced or chopped)
   splash of water

Cook until lightly softened.
Mix the following in a bowl and then add it to the pan.

   1 tablespoon tomato paste (mixed with 3 tablespoons of water)
   1 pinch basil
   1 pinch oregano
   1 pinch garlic (or 1 fresh clove)

Balance on one foot and stir the following into the pan

   2 tablespoons lowfat cottage cheese
   1/3 cup cooked short grain brown rice

Balance on the other foot and stir until the flavors dance!

# ☀ BRITTANY'S FAV "TACO THING"

*Servings: 1*
*Per serving: 282 cal, 30g Protein, 30g Carbohydrate, 5g Fat, 4g Fiber*

With care, toss the following in a medium-heat pan.
Or stir it all into a 'to go' container to heat on the road.

    3 ounces of cooked lean beef, sliced small
                    (or ground eye of round)
    ¼ small onion (chopped)
    1 tablespoon tomato paste
    2 tablespoons salsa
    1 pinch chili powder
    ½ cup water
    1 pinch of low sodium taco seasoning
    1/3 cup cooked brown rice
    ¼ cup corn
    squeeze of fresh lime (optional)

*Named after my step-daughter, she always asks for it by name.*

TIP
If you want to add more carbohydrate energy..try rolling
this mixture into a Tortilla with some lettuce.

If you want more fibrous carbohydrate throw a scoop of
"Taco Thing" on top of a lettuce salad.  Add an optional
scoop of sour cream or plain yogurt.

NOTE
I usually multiply this recipe to make several meals and
then separate it into containers for later. The spices are
enhanced that much more when you leave it sit for a while!

# ☀ CHILI....OLD FAITHFUL

*Servings: 1*
*Per serving: 284 cal, 35g Protein, 31g Carbohydrate, 5g Fat, 9g Fiber*

With care, toss the following in a medium-heat pan.
Or stir it all into a 'to go' container to heat on the road.

  3 ounces of cooked lean beef (ground eye of round)
  ½ cup kidney beans (if canned: drain & rinse)
  2 tablespoons tomato paste (mix with ½ cup water)
  ½ sm-med green bell pepper (diced)
  1 pinch chili powder (to taste)
  dash tobasco (to taste)
  1 splash worcheshire
  1 pinch garlic powder or fresh clove
  1 dash black pepper
  1 dash preferred sweetener

*I grew up in the Canadian Rockies....and there's nothing like a
good bowl of chili after playing outside on a cold winter day!*

NOTE
If you don't have the pre-cooked ingredients ready just
start with everything raw and cook it in a big pot or slow
cooker for as long as you like....the longer you simmer,
the more spicy it will become!

# ☀ INSTANT BARLEY SOUP

*Servings: 1*
*Per serving: 329 cal, 32g Protein, 28g Carbohydrate, 9g Fat, 7g Fiber*

With care, toss the following in a medium-heat pan.
Or stir it all into a 'to go' container to heat on the road.

    3 ounces of cooked lean beef (ground eye of round)
    ½ cup barley (cooked)
    1 long green onion (snipped)
    1 cup shredded cabbage or coleslaw dry mix
    1 cup water
    1 pinch defatted, low-sodium chicken or beef powder
    1 pinch basil
    1 tablespoon hemp seeds
    1 dash black pepper

NOTE
I don't usually have barley prepared all the time… so I will
often make this recipe much bigger and store it for later.

# ❰ ITALIAN FLAVORED BEEF

*Servings: 1*
*Per serving: 314 cal, 41g Protein, 30g Carbohydrate, 4g Fat, 12g Fiber*

With care, toss the following in a medium-heat pan.
Or stir it all into a 'to go' container to heat on the road.

  3 ounces of cooked lean cut of steak (sliced)
  10 ounces of california-blend veggies
  1 tablespoon flax seeds
  ½ cup onion (chopped)
  2 tablespoons tomato paste
  1 splash rice vinegar
  2 tablespoons lowfat cottage cheese or parmasan
  1 pinch low sodium italian-blend seasoning
  1 dash dried chili peppers
  1 dash preferred sweetener

Stir and cook until blended and warm.

NOTE
This is a good recipe to multiply and store for later meals.

# 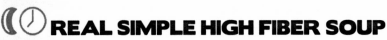REAL SIMPLE HIGH FIBER SOUP

*Servings: 8*
*Per serving: 256 cal, 25g Protein, 34g Carbohydrate, 4g Fat, 13g Fiber*
*Thanks to Denise Knorr*

Pick a BIG pot and fill it ½ full of water.
With care, toss in the following.

    20 ounces lean cut of steak (sliced) or ground eye of round
    2 pinches of black pepper
    3 pinches oregano
    3-4 cloves of garlic (minced)
    12 medium carrots (sliced)
    3 medium (5-6 cups)turnip/rutabega (cubed)
    1 medium onion (diced)
    ½ medium cabbage (shredded)

Bring to a boil while you balance on one foot and continue to stir!

Turn the heat onto simmer and leave it alone for 2-3 hours.
Go watch a movie or put on some tunes and dance.

You may want to check on the soup every once in a while and give
it a little stir.

TIP
You could also do this soup in a large crock pot.

**every baby step matters**

# 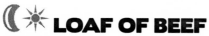 LOAF OF BEEF

*Servings: 1*
*Per serving: 313 cal, 38g Protein, 28g Carbohydrate, 6g Fat, 8g Fiber*

With care, combine the following in a bowl.

3 ounces of cooked lean beef (ground eye of round)
½ sm-med onion
2 tablespoons rolled oats
2 tablespoons low fat cottage cheese or ricotta
1 egg white or whole egg
1 squirt dijon mustard
1 dash black pepper
1 dash chili powder
1 dash oregano
1 dash preferred sweetener

Mix with your hands..play! Form a big loaf and place it into the middle of a bread pan.

Arrange the following in the pan around the loaf.

6 ounces (1 medium) carrot (sliced)

Broil in oven for 5-8 minutes.

OPTION: spread a small amount of ketchup on top.

**Tanya's Ketchup Recipe**
small can of tomato paste
1-2 splashes of apple cider vinegar
1-2 pinches of preferred sweetener
onion powder (to your taste)

# ☀ MUSHROOM BARLEY BEEF

*Servings: 1*
*Per serving: 273 cal, 29g Protein, 27g Carbohydrate, 5g Fat, 3g Fiber*


With care, toss the following in a medium-heat pan.

  3 ounces of cooked lean cut of steak (sliced)
  6 med-lrg mushrooms (sliced or not)
  ¼ sm. onion (chopped)
  ½ cup of water

Cook until most of the water has evaporated.
Add the following, cover and let simmer for a few minutes.

  ½ cup cooked barley or couscous or millet
  1 pinch low sodium bbq seasoning (ms. dash)
  1 splash red wine vinegar
  squeeze of fresh lemon or lime (optional)

Balance on one foot and stir until blended and warm.

# 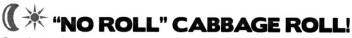 "NO ROLL" CABBAGE ROLL!

*Servings: 1*
*Per serving: 303 cal, 32g Protein, 35g Carbohydrate, 4.5g Fat, 9g Fiber*

For a couple minutes, boil 2 cups cabbage (cut or shredded) - not long, just enough to slightly soften.

Mix the following in a bowl and then stir it into the cabbage pot (drain the water first).

    3 ounces of cooked lean beef (chopped small)
                or ground eye of round
    ¼ small onion (chopped)
    ½ med tomato (diced)
    2 tablespoons tomato paste
    1 dash preferred sweetener
    ¼ cup water
    1 squirt mustard
    1 dash black pepper
    1/3 cup cooked brown rice
    1 splash rice vinegar

Let simmer for a couple of minutes.

*Unlike traditional "all day event" cabbage rolls...this one only takes a few minutes to throw together.*

TIP
I usually make 5 times the amount in a big pot, then separate it into 5 equal containers.

# 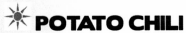 POTATO CHILI

*Servings: 1*
*Per serving: 295 cal, 30g Protein, 37g Carbohydrate, 4.5g Fat, 6g Fiber*

With care, toss the following in a medium-heat pan.
Or stir it all into a 'to go' container to heat on the road.

> 3 ounces of cooked lean beef (chopped) or ground eye of round
> 3 ounces of cooked potato (cubed)
> 2 tablespoons tomato paste
> 3 ounce cooked carrot (sliced)
> dashes chili powder (to taste)
> tobasco (to taste)
> 1 splash worcheshire
> 1 teaspoon vinegar
> 1 dash preferred sweetener
> ¼ cup water

Stir and cook until blended and warm.

NOTE
*If you don't have the pre-cooked ingredients ready just start with everything raw and cook it in a big pot or slow cooker for as long as you like….the longer you simmer, the more spicy it will become!*

*Play with your spices…be free! Find what tantalizes your taste buds…a dash here & a blend there will make a difference.*

**every baby step matters**

# ☀🕐 PREPARED CHILI

*Servings: 7*
*Per serving: 218 cal, 25g Protein, 24g Carbohydrate, 4g Fat, 6g Fiber*

With care, toss the following in a large pot on medium-heat.

1 pound cooked lean ground eye of round beef
1 small can of tomato paste
1 medium tomato (diced)
1 cup water
¼ cup rice vinegar
1 medium green pepper (diced)
1 medium onion (diced)
1 tablespoon chili powder (or to taste…the spice gets hotter the longer you simmer the chili)
3-4 cloves of garlic (sliced)
1 teaspoon black pepper
splash of worcestershire sauce
1 cup frozen corn kernels
2 cups kidney beans

Occasionally stirring, notice when the mixture begins to bubble.

Turn the heat to simmer and leave it alone for about an hour. You may want to stir it every once in a while.

NOTE
***If you use uncooked kidney beans:** DO THIS FIRST… soak them over night in a bowl with water 3 inches HIGH-ER than the beans. The next day boil the beans in that SAME water for 1 to 2 hours (until beans are soft). THEN drain and rinse before adding to the chili. YES, it is a lot of extra work, BUT it might save you from excess farting for the next couples days!*

# ✺ QUICK TOMATO BEEF N' RICE

*Servings: 1*
*Per serving: 298 cal, 32g Protein, 29g Carbohydrate, 6g Fat, 4g Fiber*

With care, toss the following in a medium-heat pan.
Or stir it all into a 'to go' container to heat on the road.

    3 ounces of cooked lean cut of steak (sliced)
    ½ cup cooked brown rice
    1 tablespoon tomato paste
    1 tablespoon vinegar
    ¼ cup water
    1 dash preferred sweetener
    2 shakes oregano or italian spice
    1 sprinkle parm cheese
    squeeze of fresh lemon or lime

Stir and cook until blended and warm.

# ◖ SIMPLE BEEF & CABBAGE

*Servings: 1*
*Per serving: 232 cal, 28g Protein, 22g Carbohydrate, 4.5g Fat, 8g Fiber*

With care, toss the following in a medium-heat pan.
Or stir it all into a 'to go' container to heat on the road.

    3 ounces of cooked lean beef (chopped)
                or ground eye of round)
    ¼ cup chopped onions
    1 cup shredded cabbage
    1 large carrot (shredded)
    dash cayenne pepper
    pinch of fresh or dried parsley
    1/8 tsp black pepper

Stir and cook until blended and warm.

# ☀ SPICY BEEF RICE

*Servings: 1*
*Per serving: 277 cal, 29g Protein, 28g Carbohydrate, 6g Fat, 4g Fiber*

With care, toss the following in a medium-heat pan with a splash of water.

    3 ounces of cooked lean cut of steak (sliced)
    ½ small to medium green pepper (chopped)
    1 sprig long green onion (snipped)
    1 dash black pepper
    1 dash crushed chili peppers or fresh thai peppers (really spicy)
    squeeze of fresh lemon or lime

Balance on one foot and stir until the flavors dance!

Serve with:

    ½ cup cooked rice

# ☀ STEAK & FRIES

*Servings: 1*
*Per serving: 263 cal, 28g Protein, 29g Carbohydrate, 4g Fat, 1g Fiber*

With care, heat oven and spray broiler-pan rack with oil.
Rub cajun spice onto:

   3-4 ounces raw lean cut steak (sliced in strips)

Boil the following until tender.

   4oz potato or yam (cut in fry strips or disks)

Broil potatoes and steak strips in oven for about 10-15 minutes, turning over at about ½ way.

# ☾ STRINGY VEGGIE WITH BEEF (FAST!)

*Servings: 1*
*Per serving: 288cal, 37g Protein, 23g Carbohydrate, 4.3g Fat, 8g Fiber*

With care, toss the following in a medium-heat pan.
Or stir it all into a 'to go' container to heat on the road.

   3 ounces of cooked lean cut of steak (sliced)
   1 cup frozen peas
   3 tablespoons 1% cottage cheese
   2 shakes black pepper

Stir and cook until blended and warm.

# ((◷ ZUCCHINI STEW

*Servings: 4*
*Per serving: 189 cal, 25g Protein, 8g Carbohydrate, 6g Fat, 2g Fiber*

With care, toss the following into a pot and bring to a boil.

  20 ounces of raw lean cut steak (sliced or cubed)
  2 large green zucchini (peeled & diced)
  1 medium onion (diced)
  1 medium tomato (chopped)
  1 cup corn kernels
  3 cloves of garlic (sliced)
  2 pinches of cummin
  2 pinches of cayenne pepper
  2 sprigs of fresh cilantro
  4 cups of water
  1 cup unsweetened, lite coconut milk

Balance on one foot and stir for a couple of minutes and then reduce the heat to simmer.

Let sit for an hour or two or three.

Keep checking the taste and adding spices if you wish.

Separate the stew into 4 equal containers.

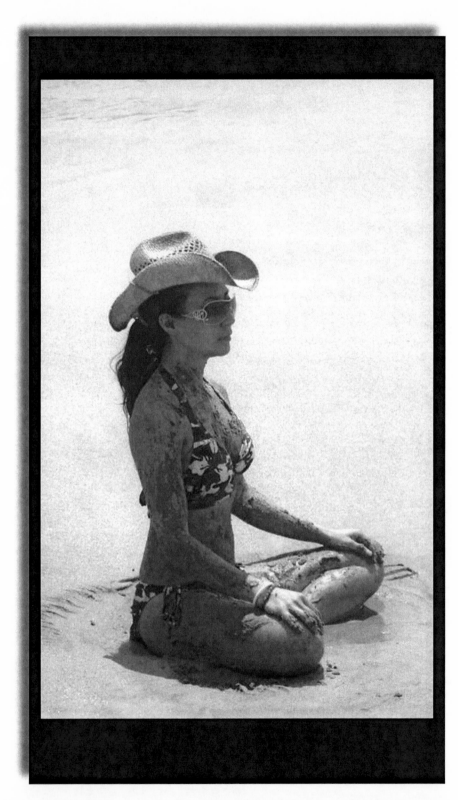

# BodyArtist

## Dr. Amanda Diep BSc., BCom., T.C.M.D.

Traditional Chinese Medical Doctor
Professional Bikini Model

I was quite an ill individual who ceased to have faith in allopathic medicine.  So, I tapped "mother nature's natural pharmacy" and exercise to find my way back to optimal health. And did I stop there? No.

I challenged myself to be in the best shape I could be - to hopefully be an example to all - that someone can actually leave the hospital (all drugged up) to then recover and work toward stage performance as a FAME Pro Bikini Model!!

I realized how blessed I am, so I'm competing on stage and using this spotlight to bring attention to one of my passions, humanitarian work. One of the non-profit organizations that I am so proud to associate with is Ministro Humanitarian Foundation.

My degrees say that I am a doctor in various areas, while my heart and soul say that I'm a humanitarian and that I'm in LOVE with life, each and everyday!

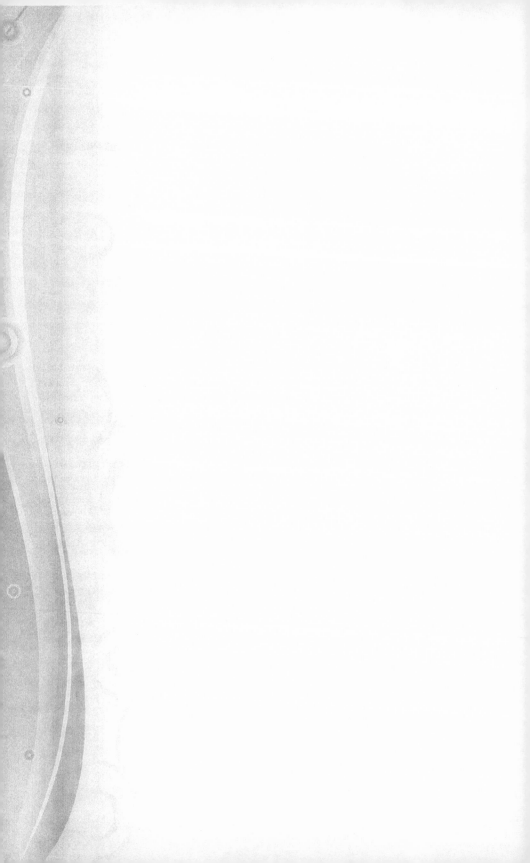

# What to do with:
# SALAD AND COLD STUFF
# meals for hot sunny days

## Lean Cuts of Beef
(sirlion or inside round)

## Poultry
(chicken and turkey breast)

## Eggs
(fresh or liquid whites)

## Fish
(tuna and cod... mostly)

# 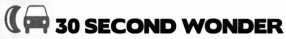 30 SECOND WONDER

*Servings: 1*
*Per serving: 127 cal, 20g Protein, 12g Carbohydrate, 0.3g Fat, 4g Fiber*

Playfully toss the following into a container, balance on one foot and stir!

½ can of tuna (canned in water or fresh)
3 tablespoons of salsa
couple handfuls (3-4 cups) of mixed salad greens

# ( BEEF WITH COLORFUL SALAD

*Servings: 1*
*Per serving: 336 cal, 33g Protein, 37g Carbohydrate, 9g Fat, 12g Fiber*

With care, mix the following in your favorite salad bowl.

3oz of lean cut of steak (cooked and sliced)
couple handfuls of fresh salad greens
½ handful of purple cabbage
1 handful of raw beats (peeled & chopped)
½ medium cumcumber (chopped)
1 small carrot (chopped)
½ red bell pepper (sliced)
½ yellow bell pepper (sliced)
½ orange bell pepper (sliced)
½ handful of sprouts
3 green olives (optional)
½ handful of chopped fresh herbs (i like basil or cilantro)

Use the following to make the dressing.

1 teaspoon of oil (hemp, udo's, olive, or grapeseed)
1 squirt of bragg's liquid amino acids or low sodium soy sauce
1 squeeze of lime juice
1 squirt of apple cider vinegar

NOTE
Considering the variety of ingredients in this recipe, it may be helpful to multiply the salad by 4-5 times and store it in the fridge.

#  CHICKPOTATO CUCUMBER SALAD

*Servings: 1*
*Per serving: 288 cal, 30g Protein, 27g Carbohydrate, 6.5g Fat, 2g Fiber*

With care, mix the following in a bowl.

- 3 oz chicken breast (cooked and diced)
- 3 oz or one small potato or yam (boiled and cubed)
- 5 oz or 1/3 of a cucumber (diced)
- 1 tablespoon reduced fat mayo
- 1 squirt worchestershire sauce
- 1 squirt bragg's amino acids
- 1 pinch fresh basil
- 1 dash black pepper

That's it. DONE!

> TIP
> Tastes even better after it has chilled in the fridge.

# ☾ CREAMY CHICK & SALSA SALAD

*Servings: 1*
*Per serving: 201 cal, 29g Protein, 14g Carbohydrate, 3.3g Fat, 4g Fiber*
*Thanks to Angela Tardiff*

With care, mix the following in a bowl.

> 2 oz or ½ chicken breast half (cooked and diced)
> ¼ cup 1% cottage cheese
> 2 tablespoons salsa

SCOOP it on to:

> 4 cups fresh mixed salad greens

That's it. DONE!

# ❨ FAST CABBAGE VINAIGRETTE

*Servings: 1*
*Per serving: 238 cal, 30g Protein, 16g Carbohydrate, 6g Fat, 8g Fiber*

*Thanks to Kiyomi Shigemi*

With care, mix the following in a bowl.

   3oz chicken breast half (cooked and diced)
   4 cups shredded cabbage mix

In a jar, shake the following to make a dressing.
While you're there, shake your hips too!

   2 splashes of vinegar
   1 teaspoon hemp, grapeseed, udo's or mct oil
   2 shakes of paprika
   2 shakes black pepper

# ☀ **FRUIT & FIBER CHICKEN SALAD**

*Servings: 1*
*Per serving: 494 cal, 36g Protein, 59g Carbohydrate, 14g Fat, 15gFiber*
*Thanks to Michele Theoret*

Playfully toss the following in a big bowl.

- 3 oz cooked chicken breast (chopped)
- ½ cup cooked barley
- ½ cup halved green and red grapes
- 2 tbsp chopped pecans
- 2 tbsp fat reduced mayo
- 1 squeeze lemon juice
- 2 cups lettuce
- ½ cup strawberries
- 1 tbsp flax seeds or hemp seeds

That's it. DONE!

# 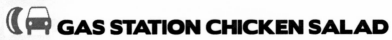 GAS STATION CHICKEN SALAD

*Servings: 1*
*Per serving: 208 cal, 30g Protein, 16g Carbohydrate, 3g Fat, 8g Fiber*

Buy:

large pre-made "to-go" salad (veggies only, no dressing)

With good intentions find a small "to go" cup to mix the following condiment counter ingredients.

2 packages of vinegar
1 package of mustard
1 package of sweetener

Pour the mixture over the salad and top with:

3oz cooked chicken breast half

NOTE
If you're traveling for the day, bring some cooked chicken with you.

Or make this a "grocery store" chicken salad and buy chicken breast from the deli. You could also buy a whole roasted chicken, eat the breast meat and share the rest with someone who likes drumsticks and wings.

**every baby step matters**

# ☾ GREEK SALAD

*Servings: 1*
*Per serving: 301 cal, 33g Protein, 24g Carbohydrate, 9g Fat,. 10g Fiber*
*Thanks to Michele Theoret*

Playfully toss the following in a big bowl.

    4 oz cooked shrimp
    2 cups romaine (chopped)
    ½ red pepper (sliced)
    ½ green pepper (sliced)
    ¼ cucumber (chopped)
    4 olives (sliced)
    1 oz light feta
    1 tbsp greek or mediterranean vinaigrette

That's it. DONE!

> TIP
> Also try cottage cheese or chicken instead of shrimp.

#  GREEN AND KIDNEY BEAN SALAD

*Servings: 1*
*Per serving: 350 cal, 37g Protein, 40g Carbohydrate, 7g Fat, 11g Fiber*

Playfully toss the following in a big bowl.

3 oz or small chicken breast half(cooked and diced)
½ cup kidney beans (drained and rinsed)
1 cup frozen cut green beans (thawed)
1 clove garlic (diced)
½ green bell pepper (sliced)
¼ small purple onion (sliced)
3 cherry tomatoes (halved)
2 splashes red wine vinegar..or just red wine
1 splash of bragg's amino acids
2 pinches fresh basil

That's it. DONE!

TIP
Tastes even better after it has sat in the fridge for a while!

# ☀🚗 IN THE VAN: TUNA SALAD

*Servings: 2*
*Per serving: 322 cal, 42g Protein, 30g Carbohydrate, 3.5g Fat, 5g Fiber*

Pull up to the next grocery store and buy the following.

- 1 can of tuna (canned in water or fresh)
- 2 small nonfat plain yogurts
- 1 mini-box of raisins
- 2 handfuls of bulk salad greens

Ask the deli for an empty 'to go' cup or salad container.
Stir everything together and eat!

# ☾ LETTUCE BEEF BOATS

*Servings: 1*
*Per serving: 254 cal, 37g Protein, 11.5g Carbohydrate, 4g Fat, 4g Fiber*

Wash and separate:

   4 full romaine leafs (boats)

Spread the following over the leaves:

   cayenne pepper
   2 tablespoons fat free cream cheese

Top with:

   3 ounces of cooked lean cut of steak (sliced)
   4 cherry or grape tomatoes (sliced in half)

TIP
Works great for guest appetizers.

**every baby step matters**

# (( 🚗 LOGUE INSPIRED FISH SALAD

*Servings: 1*
*Per serving: 180 cal, 32g Protein, 12g Carbohydrate, 0.6g Fat, 4g Fiber*

In a jar, shake the following to make a dressing.
While you're there, shake your hips too!

> couple splashes of rice vinegar
> preferred sweetener (to taste)
> dillweed
> lemon juice

Pour it over top:

> 4 cups fresh salad greens
> 4 oz cooked cod or tuna

NOTE
Donna Logue (professional IFBB bodybuilder) shared the idea of mixing vinegars with sweeteners for a simple salad dressing. Try it with different types of vinegars, spices, and salads - your options are endless.

This is only one example.

# ☀ OPEN FACE FISH & RICE CAKES

*Servings: 1*
*Per serving: 190 cal, 20g Protein, 17g Carbohydrate, 3.5g Fat, 1g Fiber*


With care, mix the following in a bowl.

½ can of tuna or 3 oz cooked white fish
1 tablespoon fat reduced mayo
1 teaspoon relish
handful of fresh salad greens or sprouts

Scoop it on to:

2 plain unsalted rice cakes

# ✳ REAL SIMPLE TUNA RICE SALAD

*Servings: 1*
*Per serving: 209 cal, 22g Protein, 29g Carbohydrate, 1g Fat, 4g Fiber*
*Thanks to Jackie Blackwater*

With care, mix the following in a bowl.

½ can tuna (canned in water or fresh)
1 tablespoon fat reduced mayo
2 dashes black pepper
½ cup cooked rice

Scoop on top of:

4 cups fresh mixed salad greens

# ( RED BELL PEPPER SALAD

*Servings: 1*
*Per serving: 240 cal, 35g Protein, 19g Carbohydrate, 5g Fat, 6g Fiber*

With care, blend the following until smooth.


½ tomato (chopped)
¼ cup non fat yogurt
splash of lemon juice or squeeze of fresh lemon
pinch of garlic powder

In a large bowl, playfully toss the following.

the blended mixture from above
3 oz or small chicken breast half(cooked and diced)
4 cups fresh salad greens
1 red bell pepper (sliced or diced)


TIP
For small portion recipes, hand-blenders are super easy to use and to clean - just run under the tap, wipe and dry.

# ☾ REFRESH! TURKEY-CRAN SALAD

Servings: 1
*Per serving:* 291 cal, 36.5g Protein, 20g Carbohydrate, 6.5g Fat, 5g Fiber

With care, blend the following until smooth.

   1 teaspoon hemp, grapeseed, or mct oil
   1/8 cup rice vinegar
   1 tablespoon fat free cream cheese

Playfully toss the following in a big bowl.

   the blended mixture from above
   3 oz turkey (cooked and diced)
   4 cups fresh salad greens
   1 roma or small tomato (sliced)
   1 tablespoon dried cranberries
   1 handful of chopped fresh basil

TIPS
Try this one with barbequed chicken too.

For small portion recipes, hand-blenders are super easy to
use and to clean - just run under the tap, wipe and dry.

# ☾ ROMAINE FISH BOATS

*Servings: 1*
*Per serving: 336 cal, 39g Protein, 23g Carbohydrate, 9.5g Fat, 10g Fiber*

Wash and separate and pat dry:

4-5 full romaine leafs (boats)

Spread the following over the leaves:

1 tablespoons fat free cream cheese

In a bowl, mix the following and scoop into romaine boats:

4oz of cooked cod
½ of small or ¼ of medium avacado (sliced)
1 x-small zuchinni (chopped)
1-2 button mushrooms (chopped)
your favorite spices

# ☀ SOUTHERN SHRIMP SALAD

*Servings: 1*
*Per serving: 535 cal, 40g Protein, 59g Carbohydrate, 17g Fat, 16g Fiber*
*Thanks to Michele Theoret*

Playfully toss the following in a big bowl.

  4 oz cooked shrimp
  ½ of small or ¼ of medium avacado (sliced)
  2 romma tomatoes (diced)
  1 tbsp each fresh diced cilantro and parsley
  black pepper to taste
  ½ cups cooked whole grain rice
  ½ cup of cooked black beans
  2 teaspoons hemp, udos, grapeseed, or olive oil
  3 tbsp balsamic vinegar

# ☾ SPINACH SALAD WITH EGG

*Servings: 1*
*Per serving: 209 cal, 22g Protein, 16g Carbohydrate, 7.5g Fat, 5g Fiber*

In a jar, shake the following to make a dressing.
While you're there, shake your hips too!

> 3 tablespoons rice vinegar
> 2 teaspoons hemp, grapeseed, udo's, or olive oil
> pinch of tarragon
> dash garlic powder
> dash paprika

Playfully toss the following in a big bowl.

> ½ cup egg beaters (cooked like scrambled eggs)
> 3 cups fresh baby spinach
> 1 cup or a handful of button mushrooms (sliced)
> ¼ small purple onion (sliced)

Top with:

> 1 tablespoon nutritional yeast

NOTE
To add a few carbohydrate/fiber grams, crumble melba
toasts to use as croutons.

**every baby step matters**

# ☾ SUPER FAST CHICK/CHEESE SALAD

*Servings: 1*
*Per serving: 224 cal, 26g Protein, 10g Carbohydrate, 9.5g Fat, 3g Fiber*


Playfully toss the following in a big bowl.

> 2 oz or ½ small chicken breast half(cooked and diced)
> 4 cups or a couple big handfuls of mixed salad greens
> 2 tablespoons 1% cottage cheese
> 2 teaspoons hemp, grapeseed, udo's or olive oil

That's it. DONE!

TIP
Try shaking your chicken in your favorite spice! I like chili powder or cayenne pepper.

# 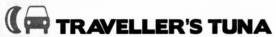 TRAVELLER'S TUNA

*Servings: 2*
*Per serving: 185 cal, 18g Protein, 9.5g Carbohydrate, 8.6g Fat, 5g Fiber*

Pull up to the next grocery store and buy the following.

- 1 can of tuna (canned in water)
- 1 small ripe avocado
- 1 cucumber

Ask the deli for an empty 'to go' cup or salad container or always keep a travel container with you.

With care, smoosh the tuna and avocado.

With your handy utility knife (every seasoned traveler has one), carve pieces of the cucumber into the mix. DONE! Enjoy!

# ☀ TUNA AND OATS...GIVE IT A TRY

*Servings: 1*
*Per serving: 351 cal, 43g Protein, 28g Carbohydrate, 9g Fat, 13g Fiber*

Balance on one foot, and stir the following in a big bowl.

1 can tuna (canned in water)
1/3 cup dry rolled oats (cook or soak in some water)
½ cup or handful of mushrooms (chopped)
1 pinch of fresh cilantro
2 teaspoons hemp, grapeseed, udo's, or olive oil
shake of black pepper

3 cups of mixed salad greens
squeeze of fresh lemon

With care, MIX together the first set of ingredients then scoop on to salad and top with squeeze of lemon.

# ☾ TUNA SWEET BROCCOLI SLAW

*Servings: 1*
*Per serving: 220 cal, 24g Protein, 13g Carbohydrate, 8g Fat, 7g Fiber*

In a jar, shake the following to make a dressing.
While you're there, shake your hips too!

  1 teaspoon hemp, grapeseed, udo's, or olive oil
  1 splash apple cider vinegar
  1 pinch of perferred sweetener
  1 dash of cinnamon

Playfully toss the following in a big bowl.

  your dressing
  ½ can  tuna (canned in water)
  8 oz or 2 handfuls of broccoli slaw
  1 tablespoon hemp seeds (hearts)

# ☀ **TUNA & PEA & RICE SALAD**

*Servings: 1*

*Per serving: 385 cal, 49g Protein, 45g Carbohydrate, 2g Fat, 11g Fiber*

Balance on one foot and stir the following in a big bowl.

  1 can  tuna (canned in water)
  1/3 cup cooked brown rice
  ½ cup frozen peas (thawed)
  1 long green onion or scallion (chopped)
  ¼ cup non fat plain yogurt
  2 pinches dry mustard powder
  splash of rice vinegar

Playfully toss the following in a big bowl.

  3 cups fresh salad greens
  1 stalk celery
  1 squeeze of fresh lemon

Top with:

  1 tablespoon nutritional yeast

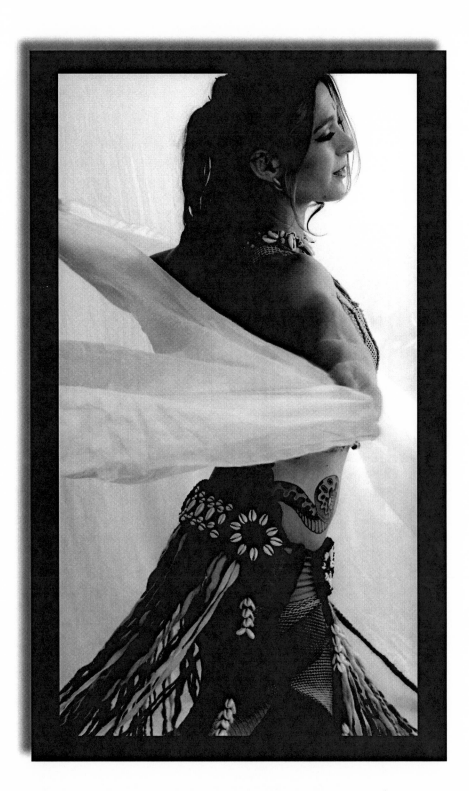

# BodyArtist

## Sami'Te

Fusion Bellydance, Fire Dance, Aerial Arts, Yoga
www.samiterocks.com

I want people to feel inspired ... to free their spirit...to grow in every direction. Dance is an expression of the heart and soul. Truly magnificent performers dance from this place.

Fusion Bellydance aims to shift paradigms...transcending the limitations of body consciousness and opening to a realm greater than ego. This realm touches the soul of any audience, inspiring people to remember the passion that burns within.

My main message is that Bellydance is a beautiful and rich artform that can be enjoyed by any body regardless of gender, age, height, weight, color, or sexual preferance. The aim of my classes is to empower the student to utilize and accentuate the gifts of their own incredible body in an environment that supports creative and spiritual growth through movement.

Blessings Be.

# Index: Vegetarian and Vegan

# Index: Meaty Meals

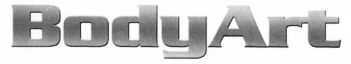

www.bodyartmotion.com

**BodyArt Motion offers private consulting, courses and educational materials for alignment, strength, nutrition and wellness with a priority to deepen self-awareness. Our intent is to simplify complex formulas into highly-functional programs that are easy-to-follow and bring into your daily life.**

**BodyArt Motion has friends in many places from fitness models on magazine covers to yoga scholars in ashrams. Whether in fight cages or belly dancing under the moon, one common thread we all share is a desire to be strong healthy and free using our body as medium to know and express ourselves. We aim to reach beyond temporary results that wear you down and extreme diets that starve the soul. BodyArt is what you sculpt for yourself emotionally and physically. It is a mind-body-soul journey that starts with how you relate with yourself – how you feel – with the aim to shift suboptimal behaviors/patterns to better serve you.**

**The foundation of our method roots from Tanya Lee's original consulting process for transformational makeovers. Today, our team continues to inspire people from all walks of life with our best selling BodyArt Cookbook and unique exercise systems: PowerAlign Yoga and Posture, GoGoBelly Dance Fitness and GZeroCore Athletic Conditioning.**

**BodyArt Cookbook Authorship**
Authored by Tanya Lee (conceived, researched, written)
Amplified by Wolfdaddy (copyedits, art direction, mantras)

**Thanks**
All authors/creators have been inspired by forces and people that flow in and out of their lives. I thank all my teachers, mentors, associates and students who taught me through what they knew and modeled as well as what they did not.

Also, I thank you, the reader! Not only for your support in purchasing the book, but also in the understanding that just by reading, feeling, and taking action based on the insights made simple within these pages, you become the author of your own body transformation. And in that metamorphosis, you will carry positive change into the world to inspire many others.

**Special Thanks**
To our mothers Andrea and Yolanda for supporting anything we choose to do with more trust than hard ass fathers seem able to source. To Yolanda for her knowledge of english grammar and eagle-eye pre-press check v5.1. To all three fathers: David, Erich, and Bob who reliably play a tough love financial advisory role.

**Global Credit**
The author's process, perspectives, phrasing, and presentation since apr2006 have been Wolfdaddy amplified. His way of being and his magic presence are truly inspirational.

**Photo Credits**
Cover photo by Ken Balaz and Tanya Lee.
Photographers and models: Kim Asburn, Dave Brown, Geordie Day, Jay "dooms" Day,

Amanda Diep, Dave Ford, Todd Ganci, Terry Goodlad, John Gordon, Christy Greene, Rachel Ibbison, Lorne Kemmet, Kristi Lees, Brittany Mein, Lea Newman, SamiTe, Gordon J Smith, Eva Sefcova, Doug Schidner, Sami Vaskola, Inga Yandell.

## Mentionable Credits

The meals in this book are designed around macronutrient ratio guidelines which have been available to bodybuilders, fitness models and athletes for decades. My journey into this and other knowledge (including a broad spectrum of food related topics) has been activated and inspired by the teachings and suggestions of many, and in particular a few special influences. Just because I credit main sources of influence does not mean that Tanya or BodyArt 100% agree with the claims/theories/institutes/publications listed below.

- body sculpting macronutrient ratios and food types have been inspired by the 1990's work of Bill Phillips (billphillips.com), 1999-2003 bodybuilding/fatloss work of Donna/Brian Logue (bodyby24-7.com), 1999-2003 fatloss/musclegain work of John Parrillo (parrillo.com), and 1993-2006 athletic performance nutrition work of Dr. Micheal Colgan (colganinstitute.com).

- wholistic food/cooking/yoga 2001 awareness focus with Bryan Kest (poweryoga.com), and 2003-2004 conscious cooking and meditation apprenticeship with Lerrita Rubinoff of Lotus Yoga Studio.

- core base micro/macronutrients inspired by the 2005 broadband studies of Wolfgang & Noel aka The Oracle Alchemist

## Unauthorized Recapitulation

The team at BodyArt Fitness dedicates their lives to the advancement of this work. Hours are spent cross-examining our own models/theories in relation to others that we include in our objective analysis in order to bring you the bares-bones break-down fundamentals.

We offer our greatest gifts to you through our consultations and publications which are always designed with the intention to benefit you.

The wisdom woven between every phrase/graphic and technique/modality is not offered to anyone to reposition as their own, directly or indirectly without our knowledge. If you would like to work with our team, co-create or evolve your own brand of BodyArt, we offer various ways we can work together.

## Authorized Reproduction

This is how you can support our mission and sustain our ability to stay on the blazing arrowhead.

All the graphics, phrases, insights, interpretations, philosophy, concepts and ideas embedded in our products are copyrighted original designs. We reserve all rights inherent yet law and ethics has never stopped the "borrowing" of ideas.

We want you to use and reuse our ideas in ways that can benefit all parties. We encourage structured recycling of our material in ways that sustain/honor the original context, as well as the commitment, energy and focus investments of key authors/inventors.

If you are an author or consultant in this area of health/fitness than know that we want you to reuse and recycle our work in yours, in its original context, accurately framed in a way that is appropriate with credit and includes our URL (www.bodyartmotion.com). So if you spin/recycle the work keep us in the loop.

E-mail: info@bodyartmotion.com

# BodyArt Motion

## info@bodyartmotion.com

### Email Our Team
When you email us, be sure to include the book's title as well as your name. We will review/share your comments with the authors and editors.

### My Bad Ass Body!
Whether you are a mom or everyday Joe, a body model, ultimate fighter, or just an Olympian, should you experience dramatic body changes feel free to share your success story and/or photos.

### Excellent Articles/Studies
If you write or find articles that you think in some way relate to our work including claims that either support or challenge it, please paste its content into an email to us and include the web address or the book/page.

### BodyArt Workshops with Tanya
If your studio would like to host/sponsor a BodyArt weekend workshop with Tanya, please contact us for more details.

### Photo Talent Development
Always artfully experimenting, BodyArt aims to work with upcoming models, fashion designers and creative photographers. Serious inquiries and professional protocols only.

### Nomadic Lab Product Testing Opportunities
We invite select producers to submit their best core fitness-nutrition-health products to our 3rd-party review as we proceed to evaluate and ultimately find what best aligns with our total solutions. The winning line-up will be featured in our books and consulting programs.

### Error/Correction Invitation
If you find typos or what you feel is a point of error, please feel encouraged to call our attention to it and/or submit corrections to our team. Earn yourself a shopping credit!

# Earn Store Credit!

Tell us how Tanya and BodyArt influenced your journey.
We want to know more about you!

Tell us if you are:
- performer dancer athlete model teacher author
- role model in the community
- military, police, fire, rescue
- big shot executive
- inspiring person
- studio owner
- busy mom
- celebrity

ONE QUICK STEP
Photocopy this page.
Fill it out and mail to:  BodyArt
Box 397, Cremona, Alberta Canada T0M 0R0

*Note: none of your personal information will be published or shared with anyone
without your prior knowledge.*

**BodyArt Welcomes Your Feedback**
The more you share with us the more valuable it is to us in understanding who
uses our products and how best to evolve our services.  Know your customers.
Serve them better.

   full name
   biz name
   city
   email

1. How did you hear about BodyArt?


2. What is your primary goal with our products?

*get strong    get toned    look better naked    feel more confident
increase body awareness    other:*


3. Do you teach or hold titles in performance, athletics, modeling, or other movement disciplines? Please list.


4. Any other labels that apply such as professional, executive, doctor, busy parent, college student?


5. What do you find most useful about BodyArt products/services.

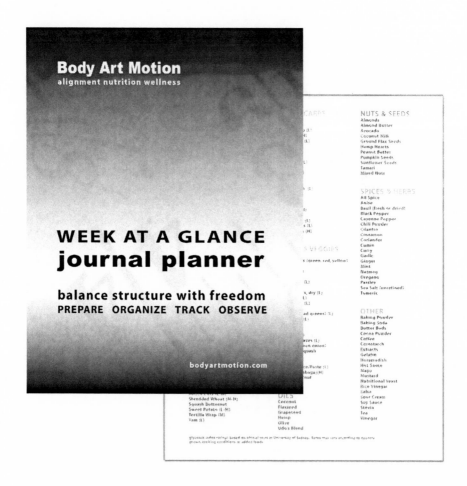

# BodyArt Journal Planners
# Customized For Your Journey

- start anytime of the year
- 3 month format with goal setting & reflection
- two versions: day at a glance & week at a glance

www.bodyartmotion.com

# Casting-Call :: Ongoing Model Search

We want to promote you by featuring your photos, hosting your website and inviting you to projects and photoshoots!

BodyArt Model Search is for women who were born for the spotlight, and who value a strong healthy body. To us, healthy means you have meat on your bones, try your best to embody your values, and know in your gut that feeling comfortable in your body is a journey of heart and soul.

So send us your best photos and a few sentences on what you value most and what inspires you to move.

Watch for these amazing women in BodyArt books and on bodyartmotion.com. If you think you, or someone you know, would be a great BodyArt Model and would benefit from the perks below, then send us your best photos and writing.

info@bodyartmotion.com

All Models Receive:
1. FREE affiliate website hosting for one year ($100 value)
2. Discount on business solutions by Vision2Bank
3. Feature photos in BodyArt publications
4. FREE BodyArt Cookbook

--------------------------------------------------------------------------------

**MAJOR SPONSOR OF BODYART CASTING-CALLS**

Vision 2 Bank  Business Start-up Solutions
For Artists, Athletes, Dancers and Models
Make a living doing what you love!  Sculpt your core offering.
Produce high-function creative business solutions.

www.vision2bank.com

# *Seminars Courses Workshops*

Bring Tanya to your corporate event, studio, gym, retreat

*Bring our entertaining and educational mobile school to your corporate event, studio, gym, or weekend bootcamp intensive retreat. Tanya teaches BAM courses for both mainstream audiences and for fitness/wellness professionals. Ask us about affiliated credits for your professional associations.*

## POWERALIGN

PowerAlign is our core language library with exercise routines that strengthen posture, develop body-mind connection, and prepare you for safe and effective movement using internal techniques and subtle awareness.

The focus is on fundamentals needed for safe and effective exercise and general integrity for posture in motion. The purpose is to give you the confidence and essential tools needed to optimize your own practice and any group classes you visit.

## DESK JOCKEY RESCUE

PowerAlign techniques applied for desk jockeys, office staff, long commuters, frequent fliers and jet set execs. Benefit from basic posturing techniques, core stability, stretching, low back stability, and shoulder/neck relaxation.

Tanya wants our posture optimized so we can better enjoy what we do - able to move through long days with grace and ease - ultimately able to handle greater stress at work. Tanya's Pinup Professor adds a humorous flare to her formal presentation, leaving her corporate audiences relaxed and engaged.

## GOGOBELLY

PowerAlign techniques applied for the motions of GoGoBelly dance. These fun and flirty drills and techniques will get your posture strong as well as feel and express your femininity.

This course is beginner level, focusing on the basics - no experience or coordination needed! Learn how to safely and effectively shimmy your hips, flirt with your shoulders, control your abdominal muscles, isolate your glutes - all while firing up hot moves and holding your space with grace.

## POWER YOGA FUSION

This fusion format yoga practice is a deep integration of various exercises, breathing techniques and meditation disciplines. Various forms of Yoga as well as Pilates are integrated in a way that honors specific essences true to each practice.

Segments are sewn together in a master sequence that follows a "spiral flow" which mimics the natural life cycle. This format is simple, clean, mainstream and inclusive of 8 essential elements: deep core integrity, spinal mobility, inner strength, energy stimulation, flow/grace, balance, equanimity and relaxing visualization.

## BAM NUTRITION AND EATING HABITS

Create a balanced relationship with food and gain awareness of macro-nutrients needed to fuel active muscles, sustainably sculpt body weight, control moods and overeating, and allow you to eat more of the foods you love.

Balance structure with freedom. Humans are too dynamic and complex to have a one size fits all approach to proper nutrition. Tanya offers inspiration and creativity as well as general guidelines and rules that have proven to act as a solid foundation you can rely upon.

## SEASONS AND CYCLES

Have you ever wondered why traditional yoga is not practiced on new and full moons, or why bodybuilders/athletes "cycle" their diet & training regimes? In this course, you will gain awareness to yearly and monthly cycles of nature and how they affect our body-mind.

Learn functional information on how to tap into the power of these cycles for physical training, rest/relaxation, mental focus and goal setting. Tanya draws from her years of Astropsychology studies as well as comparisons from basic physiology/psychology of the menstrual cycle and athletic periodization in order to show how both of these patterns correlate with sun-moon cycles.

Contact us for more information:

info@bodyartmotion.com

(403) 313-5775

# RECOGNITION

## BEHIND THE SCENES

Wizards Conjure Magic Behind The Curtain

Wolf Lawrence is a key contributor to my projects and my life.  He is one amazing dude - a broadband professor with a seasoned bullshit radar. Wolf continues to be my personal dance teacher and puzzlemaster for team BodyArt Motion. Wolfdaddy, you rock!

## www.bigwolfdaddy.com

*"Tanya combines exercise, nutrition, art, philosophy, yoga, and a search for insight to teach, touch, and inspire the rest of us."*

KEVIN MYLES  writer editor Body Sport Magazine

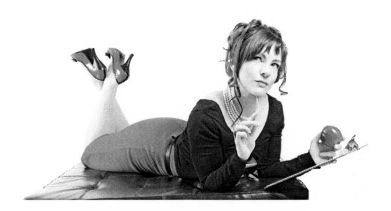

Tanya Lee is an author, educator and yoga trainer. She specializes in exercise & eating habits, posture alignment & RSI, dance-fitness and sustainable body sculpting. She is the author of the BodyArt Cookbook and Alignment Secrets, and designed the PowerAlign multi-disciplinary movement system. As a pioneer on the cutting edge, Tanya cofounded one of the first schools in Canada to combine Yoga, Pilates and Mixed Martial Arts. She was also in the champion circle for Canada's first officially sanctioned fitness model competition.

Firmly founded in the cycles of nature, Tanya's method has helped thousands of everyday people feel and look better in their bodies since 1997. Her works on nutrition and movement have been validated for over a decade by health and fitness professionals including MDs, Chiropractors, Champion Athletes, Dancers & Models, Yoga, Pilates and Rehab Specialists.

From multiple disciplines, she discovers efficient ways to approach and optimize the classics. Often sought after as "coach of coaches" and "trainer of trainers", Tanya designs advanced body-mind-emotion programs that focus on the basics with meaning and purpose. Instructors certified in her methods have gone on to coach professional sports teams, mentor fitness models, lead performance troupes and open successful studios.

Committed to her mission, Tanya stays busy translating core fundamentals of movement, nutrition and awareness into easy-to-digest layered programs, seminars, consulting and books. Unlike other lucky stars, Tanya doesn't have a kitchen staff or use ghost writers - she actually writes and assembles all her own work from her experience and case studies.

Her testimonials include victims of sciatica and low back pain, stroke, abuse and sex trauma, stress/anxiety, birthing pelvic trauma, addictive eating and body-image disorders. See how others have worked with Tanya Lee to optimize their own outlook and regime to enjoy greater success, personal discovery and self-worth.

CPSIA information can be obtained at www.ICGtesting.com
Printed in the USA
LVOW111544240212

270297LV00002B/22/P